The
Miracle
Workout

The Miracle Workout

THE

REVOLUTIONARY

3-STEP PROGRAM

FOR *YOUR*

PERFECT BODY

W. Jackson Davis, Ph.D.

ACSM-CERTIFIED HEALTH/FITNESS INSTRUCTORSM

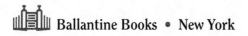 Ballantine Books • New York

Published in the United States by Ballantine Books, an imprint of The Random House Publishing Group, a division of Random House, Inc., New York.

Ballantine and colophon are registered trademarks of Random House, Inc.

Line drawings by P. T. Nunn

Library of Congress Cataloging-in-Publication Data
Davis, W. Jackson (William Jackson), 1942–
    The miracle workout : the revolutionary 3-step program for your perfect body /
by W. Jackson Davis.—1st ed.
        p. cm.
    Includes bibliographical references.
    ISBN 0-345-47080-X (alk. paper)—ISBN 0-345-47081-8 (trade : alk. paper)
    1. Physical fitness.   2. Exercise.   I. Title.
GV481.D37 2005
613.7'1—dc22   2004061681

Printed in the United States of America

Ballantine Books website address: www.ballantinebooks.com

9 8 7 6 5 4   3 2 1

First Edition

Text design by Mary A. Wirth

*Dedicated to the
remembrance of
Ian Carney*

ADVISORIES AND DISCLAIMERS

Exercise of any kind, including the Miracle Workout introduced in this book, carries inherent benefits and risks. Before you begin the Miracle Workout or any other program of exercise or change in physical activity, consult with a qualified medical professional to ensure that the benefits outweigh the risks for you. If you are pregnant, or a member of any special clinical population (chapter 9), consult with your doctor before starting this or any other fitness program. As with any exercise or diet program, if you experience any faintness, shortness of breath, pain, or other discomfort at any time, stop immediately and obtain qualified medical advice and/or assistance.

References in *The Miracle Workout* to my work with athletes at the University of California, and identification of my professional affiliation with the University, should in no case be construed as advertisement or promotion of *The Miracle Workout* or any other activity described in this book. References in *The Miracle Workout* to the University of California in no way imply that the university is involved or affiliated with, or supports, endorses, advances, recommends, or otherwise warrantees or vouches for, any aspect of the Miracle Workout or any other activity described in this book.

AUTHOR'S PATENT NOTICE

The Miracle Workout methods and related materials described in this book are proprietary inventions of W. Jackson Davis and are protected by U.S. and international copyright law as well as by one or more U.S. and/or international patent applications (Patent Pending) or patents. *Any individual who is in good health is welcomed and encouraged to practice the Miracle Workout methods and use the related workout logs, forms, and related materials published in this book, for their own personal, noncommercial purpose(s).* The Miracle Workout methods, workout logs, forms, and related materials may not be used, however, for any commercial or nonprofit purpose without the express written permission of W. Jackson Davis. Prohibited uses include, but are not limited to, performing, teaching, describing, reproducing, or distributing in any form the Miracle Workout methods, workout logs, forms, and related materials. All rights reserved.

Many mentors, teachers, coaches, workout partners, colleagues, and friends contributed to this book, directly and indirectly. These pivotal figures in my life taught, challenged, and shaped my purpose and direction in ways neither they nor I might have imagined, and this book would not have been possible without them. This book benefited also from the publications, training programs, and certification programs of the American College of Sports Medicine (ACSM), including the ACSM professionals who presented my certification workshop and made it an exciting learning experience: director Dr. Sandy Bulmer, Dr. Kathy Jankowski, John White, Dan McClure, Reneé Prosen, T. J. Hall, and Toni Bloom.

Throughout the original scientific research that underpins this book, the people of the Office of Physical Education, Recreation, and Sports (OPERS) at the University of California at Santa Cruz (UCSC) shared outstanding facilities, expertise, and resources with patience and generosity. I am particularly grateful to my collaborators, Dr. Dan T. Wood, OPERS executive director; Ryan Andrews, director of the UCSC Wellness Center and its world-class gym; and Les Elkind, MD, who heads the UCSC Student Health Services. I thank also Greg Harshaw, the university's athletic director, who helped implement this work in the athletic department; Paul Holocher, the UCSC men's soccer coach, and Michael Runeare, the UCSC women's soccer coach, for their support and assistance during training; Sarah Pinneo, who helped train the women athletes; Danielle Lewis, who helped in data acquisition; and Sonia Williams-Kelley, who was instrumental in data analysis. Numerous others aided or supported the training and research, including Tamara Chinn, James Cisneros, Laura Engelken, Dianne Fridlund, Jill Fusari, Cindy Hodges, Kathleen Hughes, Robert Irons, Camille Jarmie, Kristin Onorato, Karen

Ostermeier, Mischa Plunkett, Onelia Rodriquez, Zoe Scott, Justin Smith, and Kelly Vizcarra.

UCSC supported the work in countless ways. The Institutional Review Board administered by Caitlin Deck, Dierdre Beach, and Kata Aja oversaw the scientific research and ensured consistency with federal and state guidelines covering research on human subjects. I thank Professor Bruce Bridgeman, chair of the Human Subjects Research Committee, and committee members Les Elkind, Daniel Friedman, Dobie Jenkins, and Alice Yang-Murray, for their competent oversight and review. I am grateful for the opportunity to teach exercise physiology in the university's Discovery Seminar Series, established by Executive Vice Chancellor Dr. Lynda Goff and administered by Ken Christopher, Margie Claxton, and Greta Gil. The integration of the research in this book with the teaching of exercise physiology, and the enthusiasm and critical thinking of my students, contributed to my growth in this field.

My deepest gratitude and respect go to the student-athletes who participated as subjects in the scientific research. Their discipline and hard work helped manifest the miracles. They are: Chris Alexander, Paige Alumbaugh, Jim Anderson, Kevin Anderson, Brian Baird, Kim Bernet, Eric Bucchere, Ian Carney, Caitlin Carpenter, Dan Chamberlain, Lauren Chiodini, Ashley Cleland, Gabriel Craig, George Crocker, Sarah Dixon, Andrew Donnolly-Crocker, Fred Dreier, Erin Flynn, Courtney Frick, Kathleen Gardiner, Eric Gibbs, Bret Gravlin, Jennifer Guro, Claire Gustafson, Barr Haney, Victoria Henry, Gilad Hoffman, Joshua Holtrust, Kirstin Horn, Uilanikuulei Kaanapu, Matt King, Leanna Klistoff, Jenna Koch, Nick Kowba, Martina Kroll, Aaron Lanes, Monica Lee, Lauren Lindsay, Grant Lyon, Aaron Miyasaki, Brina Mocsny, Kurt Munoz, Kristin Parks, Lauren Philibosian, Regina Rameriz, Crystal Russo, Jaclyn Salle, Danielle Sassano, Michelle Sharman, Leah Smith, Skye Vendt-Pearse, Marisol Visalli, Ben Weston, and Ivy Whitford. Thank you, athletes! I will never forget you and your enthusiastic dedication—or, for that matter, our 6 AM workouts.

Jim Levine, of Levine Greenberg Literary Agency in New York, saw the possibilities of *The Miracle Workout* early, and his guidance helped immeasurably to bring them to life. He and his colleagues, Melynda Bissmeyer, Stephanie Rostan, and Arielle Eckstut, turned the traditional chore of publishing into a treasured source of support and friendship. Artist P. T. Nunn created the line drawings, and she and Dave Jordan designed and developed the website that accompanies this book (www.MiracleWorkout.com). Kenny Jowers, of the Physical Gym in Gualala, California, generously loaned his facilities in support of the artwork.

The professionals at Random House, including my editor Mark Tavani and Maureen O'Neal, encouraged progress in every possible way. Mark edited the book patiently and skillfully, and in the process made the writing readable. Patricia Nicolescu and Laura Jorstad also contributed critically to the editing, and Gene Myd-lowski and his talented team of designers created the attractive jacket. And special thanks to Ingrid Powell for her assistance. Helpful reviews of the manuscript came from Rebecca Davis and Will Satterthwaite. I am responsible for any remaining errors. Photography credits go to D. T. Wood, C. Helade, and Ron Bolander.

This book would not exist without the love, support, advice, and insights of my wife, Claudia Helade. She was instrumental in prompting the scientific research, provided invaluable suggestions and counsel at every stage of the project, and reviewed and vastly improved successive stages of the manuscript. Finally, to my parents, William Jackson Davis Sr. and Ruth Lorraine Lawrence Davis, thanks for everything.

W. Jackson Davis
July 2004
The Sea Ranch, California

The Miracle Workout

1

The Integrated Exercise Revolution

This book is about a revolutionary way to manage your weight, sculpt your body, and reach peak performance, all in record time. The method is proven and easy, and it works regardless of your current physical condition, age, or personal goals. It is based on a newly discovered natural approach to exercise that is in reality as old as the hills, but has been long hidden in plain sight. I call it Integrated Body Conditioning, or simply IBC.

You have already practiced elements of IBC, though you probably didn't recognize it. You did it when you were a child without giving it a second thought—you just played, and knew it was fun. You can recapture similar magic as an adult with IBC. In the process, you can work miracles with not just your body but also your mind, emotions, and spirit. This book is your performance manual for IBC, your path to the best body you can have, and, if you're ready, your ticket to a new life. IBC has changed the nature and perception of exercise for me. When you finish reading this first chapter, I think you will feel the same way, and by the time you complete your first few IBC workouts, I know you will.

A Chronicle of Miracles

Since I discovered it years ago, integrated exercise has changed my life. Because of IBC, my muscle strength and endurance at the chronological age of 62 years exceed the 90th percentile of men in the 20–29 year age group. My maximum heart rate is typical of a 35-year-old man, and my bone strength and joint function resemble those of a 45-year-old man. And trust me—I am no genetic superman. I owe this personal miracle to a workout anyone can do, at any age, and at any level.

IBC can work miracles for you, too. It will bring you to your full genetic potential with minimum pain and in the least possible time. IBC can help reduce your body weight to its optimum level without calorie-restriction diets and without drugs, with due qualifications for members of special populations (chapter 9). Put IBC together with the integrated diet (chapter 10), and miracles follow. Perhaps most important for the long term, IBC is fun. To get and stay fit for life, you've got to enjoy the process. People who try the IBC workout generally rank it as their favorite, because it's fun to do, it's energizing, and it gives you a new vitality between workouts. Once your IBC program is under way, you may feel more invigorated than you've felt in years.

IBC is energizing because it conditions all three of your body's primary energy systems—the short-term phosphorous (your biochemical first gear), medium-term anaerobic (second gear), and long-term aerobic (third gear) energy systems. IBC is an energy-conditioning approach to exercise. In the process, it also produces unprecedented results in fat loss, muscle gain, cardiovascular health, aerobic capacity, muscle strength, and muscle endurance. Controlled, randomized, and double-blind scientific experiments on college athletes at the University of California (chapter 3) show that IBC builds muscle twice as fast as the best conventional exercise prescription, and reduces fat three times faster than the best conventional exercise prescription—and all with little or no muscle soreness.

IBC is also your path to peak body flexibility. You may stretch and bend like a child again, with minimum discomfort. You can achieve these miracles for yourself anywhere you choose—indoors or out, at home or in a gym, in as little as 30 minutes per session, three times a week. Most important, IBC is thoroughly adaptable to your needs and preferences—and pocketbook. You can do the IBC workout inexpensively and with minimum equipment, and make it as easy—or as hard—as you want or require, depending on your level and goals. For example:

- If you are new to exercise and your goals are limited to losing pounds and keeping them off, feeling energetic, and being healthy and well, do the beginning (30-minute) IBC workout three or more times a week (chapter 4). It's a cinch.
- If you are already exercising and in reasonable physical shape, and your goals include top physical fitness, select the intermediate (60-minute) IBC workout (chapter 5). It's vigorous, but within the reach of most healthy people.

- If you are an advanced exerciser or athlete, and if your goals extend to peak performance, use the 90-minute-plus IBC workout (chapter 6), in combination with sport-specific training exercises (chapter 7) and a year-round program designed to peak just before your season. It's a challenge.
- If you are a member of a special population, there may be an IBC workout for you, although you may require special precautions (chapter 9).
- If you are a senior with restricted capacities, or recovering from injury or illness, there may be an IBC workout for you—if your doctor approves (chapter 9).
- If you belong to a sports team or are a coach and have the will to excel, there is an IBC program for you and your athletes (chapter 3).

IBC helped propel the University of California at Santa Cruz men's soccer team to the NCAA West Regional championship and the national championship finals two years in a row. The IBC workout is working miracles for the women's soccer team, too, and it has become the foundation for conditioning in the UCSC athletic program. It's so easy to learn, so effective and energizing, so downright exhilarating, that your days of dreading exercise are over.

How IBC Works

IBC has three primary elements:

1. **Integrate different modes of exercise into the same workout.**
   This book shows you the different modes—aerobic, resistance, flexibility—and how to assemble them into a quick, fun, highly efficient workout with simple, adaptable routines and (if you choose) user-friendly workout logs to record your progress.
2. **Exercise at a properly elevated heart rate.**
   This book shows you how to build up to that point safely, at your own pace, and determine and monitor your correct heart rate training window for optimum conditioning in light of your personal goals.
3. **Progress steadily according to how your body feels.**
   This book shows you a simple method to look within to optimize perceived exertion and minimize perceived pain while you exercise. That way, you can advance at your body's own best pace with minimum discomfort and minimum risk of injury.

Here's a preview of the IBC workout. Start with an exercise as easy as a brisk daily walk to improve your cardiovascular condition. Then use your newly empowered heart to develop the rest of your body. While your heart rate is elevated into your cardiovascular training window—we'll see exactly what that means shortly—do other kinds of exercise, such as stretching, bending, lifting, pushing, and pulling. When you do these other exercises while your heart rate is elevated, both your heart and the rest of your body develop much faster, in a mutually reinforcing growth cycle.

This first guiding principle of IBC is cardio-driving. This and several additional IBC principles and practices tap directly into biological universals (chapter 2)—the physiological common denominators of every human being. You can therefore apply them to Pilates, Spinning, Yoga, or any other exercise system. If you already have a regular exercise routine going for yourself, and if you enjoy it, a few small modifications may enable you to apply IBC principles to your current exercise program and harvest dual benefits.

The IBC program is a three-step process. Think of it as a band or orchestra with three sections. You start with the rhythm section—your heart. Cardiovascular conditioning, commonly called aerobics, is your first step on the IBC path to balanced development. Once you have attained adequate cardio condition, you add the string section—stretching and bending, or Range of Motion (ROM) exercises—to your aerobic routine. When you achieve a satisfactory measure of body flexibility, IBC adds the brass section—resistance exercise, or weightlifting. Then, and only then, your body will begin to make the soaring music that it is capable of creating and that nature intended. Once your IBC program is well under way, adjust what you eat as required to achieve your desired equilibrium body weight, following the integrated diet (chapter 10), and you'll be well along the path to realizing the fullest potential of the human body, mind, and spirit—and the integrated life.

Why Should You Bother?

Let us count the ways, starting with looking and feeling as good as you can. You will enhance your everyday coordination and balance, sleep soundly without drugs, minimize and manage everyday pain without drugs, improve your love life, and protect against injury. Research shows that regular exercise can even improve incontinence.

As we'll develop in the next chapter, your mind will benefit, too. You maximize mental acuity when you exercise regularly, you have more physical energy, and you experience more raw vitality. Regular exercise reduces depression and anxiety, which are approaching epidemic levels in this culture. Exercise even lessens the risks of contracting Alzheimer's disease, which currently afflicts four million Americans and, according to medical experts, could increase fivefold by 2050.

IBC can lessen your risk of heart disease, which kills another one in four Americans. Blood pressure is on the rise in the United States—one American in three, 60 million adults, now have high blood pressure, or hypertension, and a corresponding increased risk of cardiovascular disease. IBC can reduce blood pressure dramatically (chapter 3), without drugs and their often grisly side effects. Regular exercise is also a key to combating obesity, which according to the UN World Health Organization is now responsible for 60 percent of the 56.5 million deaths that occur around the world each year.

Regular exercise even reduces the risk of most forms of cancer, which currently kills one in four Americans. Fully one-third of all cancers in the United States are directly attributable to diet and physical activity patterns, and

> *Evidence from more than 25 research studies on humans (from different continents with different diets, ways of life, environmental circumstances, race, ethnicity and socio-economic backgrounds) . . . show a reduced risk of cancer development associated with higher levels of regular physical activity.*[1]

Regular exercise can even help you minimize the health impacts of toxins in the environment. Each of us, no matter where we live on the earth, carries an unavoidable body burden of pesticides such as DDT and other toxins, as one of the downsides of industrial civilization. IBC can help minimize the risk, because many toxins are stored in fat, and the level of these toxins in blood plasma is as much as one-third lower in people who stay lean. The intermediate and advanced IBC workouts also give you the full-body flush (chapter 5), a bath from the inside out, which helps eliminate wastes from your body.

Why should you bother? In a sentence—because IBC is fun, inexpensive, efficient, and a proven fast track to health and wellness, physical fitness, and peak performance.

The Origin of Integrated Body Conditioning

Many before me have "discovered" elements of IBC. Animals do it naturally as part of their daily existence. Children do it every day when they play. IBC is built into numerous sports, including Nordic (cross-country) skiing, all-terrain mountain biking, and Olympic wrestling, to name a few. Several exercise systems or programs also incorporate IBC elements. Circuit training was among the earliest, and still comes closest. UCLA's Professor Laurence Morehouse was on the right track a generation ago. Some elements of IBC appear in many established exercise programs, such as muscle in motion, Power Sculpting, Spinning, and the Real Simple routine. Power walking and ShapeWalking contain components of IBC, as does the HeavyHands exercise program. Some power lifters use the Westside Barbell method, which entails rapid performance of heavy weightlifting exercises. The Curves' franchise markets elements of IBC to a special population, and the U.S. military incorporates certain aspects of integrated exercise into basic training.

Elements of IBC have therefore already been applied to physical conditioning programs, although unknowingly and unsystematically. The three original contributions of this book are:

- To define the elements of IBC.
- To explore their remarkable capacities through scientific research.
- To distill the elements into a simple, efficient, and fun workout that you or your group or team can do safely, in steps, at any level, and anywhere, for a lifetime.

My personal process of exploration and discovery began with years of self-experiment using IBC, followed by scientific studies at the University of California. My colleagues and I evaluated IBC objectively, compared it with the best conventional exercise prescription, and used it to train collegiate athletes in several sports, including soccer, swimming, volleyball, tennis, and basketball. That experience helps affirm the results you can achieve with IBC.

Above all, my goal in writing this book is to make IBC accessible to all. I wrote it to show you how to harness the power of IBC in a workout that works for you—whatever your goals or current level—as a lifelong practice.

The Discovery of Integrated Body Conditioning

The IBC story begins half a century ago when, as a teenager in Silicon Valley, I started my first weightlifting program in the family garage. I continued to exercise regularly through my undergraduate years at the University of California at Berkeley, spending countless hours practicing a precursor to IBC, circuit training. I kept it going into my 30s, but then, like so many people, life and career responsibilities intervened, and regular exercise suffered.

Throughout my middle age, I exercised in fits and starts, careening in and out of physical fitness perhaps a dozen times over three decades. Over this half century, I practiced almost every exercise program ever invented, and discovered anew every excuse to avoid it. Had I known about IBC earlier, I might have avoided all that zigzagging, and I hope I can spare you the same fate. In hindsight, however, this long personal incubation, including many stops and starts, is what led me to IBC and helped me recognize it when I stumbled upon it many years ago.

It happened like this. During one of many exercise comebacks, I changed my usual sequence of exercise and started my workout with aerobics, which conditions the heart, lungs, and vascular system. The conventional wisdom of strength training in those days was to start each workout with an initial short warm-up and then move straight to weightlifting and rest between exercises. Combining aerobics with weightlifting was taboo among exercise professionals. In contrast, however, I discovered that the longer and more vigorous my warm-up, the better I felt during subsequent weight training. So my warm-up just kept getting longer. Eventually I found myself starting every workout with 30 minutes of vigorous cardio exercise, followed by weightlifting. To save time, I took no pause between the cardio machine and my first resistance (weightlifting) exercise. With my heart still racing, I moved straight to the hip machine.

That is where the miracle began. After the first few hip workouts at an elevated heart rate, my hip strength and endurance showed what appeared to be an impossible increase. Within a few months of the fastest physical progression I had ever experienced, I could effortlessly do 100 repetitions with the machine's heaviest weight—240 pounds. Most astonishing, this stunning progress occurred with no muscle soreness.

I am a scientist by training. I spent two decades researching the brain and behavior before I left the laboratory for other pursuits. My early results with IBC, however, proved anew that you can take the scientist out of the laboratory, but you can't take the laboratory out of the scientist. At that point in my exercise program, the scientist within took over. My early results with hip exercises initiated years of systematic self-experimentation in the gym, testing and retesting the hypothesis that an elevated heart rate during weightlifting produces unprecedented gains in muscle strength and endurance with little or no muscle soreness.

My legs were the next target. I moved without pause from the cardio machine to the inclined leg press sled and did leg presses at an elevated heart rate. Leg presses are one of the best all-around machine exercises, which is why they are a part of the gym IBC workout at every level (chapters 4–6). Within a few months of that simple change in exercise sequence, I leg pressed 1,200 pounds. The most I had ever managed as a graduate student in my 20s was about half that. Most surprising to me, I could not make my leg muscles sore, regardless of how hard I tried.

So far so good, but up to this point all my tests were limited to postural muscles—the slow but enduring muscles that steady us in space by chronic contraction. It was time to broaden the experiment by performing the same self-test on the pectorals (pecs), or chest muscles. Nature designed the pecs for contraction speed and strength, rather than endurance, and composed them largely of fast-twitch muscle fibers that are stronger, but fatigue faster. This would provide a new and different test of IBC.

In a few months, my Smith Rack bench press soared from 180 pounds to 300 pounds. My previous personal record, set when I was a graduate student, was 220 pounds. It appeared that this new mode of conditioning worked not only for postural muscles, but also for fast-twitch muscles. I turned next to the abdomen, whose muscles are part of the critical core that supports all other exercise. Within a few months, I did sets of 100 abdominal curl-ups or crunches on an inclined bench, alternated with a minute of cardio exercise, for hours—literally.

The conclusion appeared inescapable: To reach previously unthinkable exercise goals fast and largely without muscle soreness, keep your heart rate suitably elevated at the same time that you do other exercises, and progress at your own pace to unheard-of heights. IBC harnesses the aerobic "runner's high" and directs this rarefied physical and mental state to accelerate fat loss, muscle gain, body flexibility, and muscle strength and endurance.

I was by then convinced that IBC worked for me, but my scientific curiosity was piqued, and other explanations for my unprecedented personal results remained plausible. Perhaps I was simply reaching down deeper than I had in younger years, an unconscious last hurrah. Even if my findings were genuine, it was not clear whether they applied only to me, or if other people of different ages, races, and body types could achieve similar results. I needed evidence more persuasive than a testimonial from myself, and I could not rest until IBC had withstood the higher standard of controlled, randomized, double-blind scientific testing on a larger population of women and men.

I had worked out, off and on, for more than 30 years in the superb facilities of the Department of Physical Education, Recreation, and Sports (OPERS) at the University of California at Santa Cruz (UCSC), where I teach. I approached the OPERS director, Dr. Dan Wood, about initiating a program of scientific research on IBC. We were joined by Ryan Andrews, who runs the UCSC gym and its nationally known Wellness Program. Ryan is a doubly certified personal trainer, and early in our work together he did the IBC workout himself—the first subject besides me. He experienced rapid development from an already superb base of physical condition, providing valuable reassurance at a crucial juncture. Chapter 3 highlights the results of this scientific odyssey.

This is not, however, a scientific treatise. My goal is to bring this workout to as many people as possible, and I wrote this book as a practical owner's manual to enable you to incorporate IBC into your life. You can become fully capable in IBC, and reap all its benefits, with no scientific background whatever—or, for that matter, without any interest in or need for the science. If this describes you, skip straight to chapter 4, try the IBC workout yourself, and see what happens. You are always the best judge of what works for you.

Exercise Outside the Box

Sound science underlies IBC, but in hindsight IBC turns a great deal of conventional workout wisdom on its head. I had to let go of several basic tenets of exercise physiology and science that I had embraced over half a century of exercising, and recondition my thinking in the IBC framework. It all makes perfect biological and evolutionary sense (chapter 2).

One Program Fits All.

Conventional wisdom, for example, holds that there is no perfect workout for everyone. There is truth here. Different people like to do different things, come to exercise at different initial levels, and have vastly different exercise goals. In addition, there's the law of specificity, which dictates that any training effect is specific to the activity that produces it (chapter 7).

From a biological viewpoint, however, the fundamentals of human physiology are alike in everyone. We're all made of the same stuff, water and stardust, and have 600 muscles, 206 bones, and 100 billion nerve cells. These components of the human machine all work pretty much the same way. Biologists even have a name for it— evolutionary conservatism. If some basic biological process works a particular way in one person, or even in a squid, it probably works similarly in all people and even all living creatures. IBC addresses the biological universals of human genetics and physiology, the common denominators of human biology, like no other approach to exercise.

Less Pain, More Gain.

IBC dispels another hallowed myth of exercise that you have no doubt encountered—*No pain, no gain*. Generations of exercisers have followed this creed, though in recent years experts increasingly question it. The idea arose because conventional exercise done at high intensity makes your muscles burn and can leave you unbearably sore for the next several days with Delayed Onset Muscle Soreness (DOMS). We have all felt it—recall that weekend you played touch football or gardened all day and paid the price well into the following week with excruciating muscle soreness. IBC not only does not hurt while you're doing it, but also leaves little or no residual soreness.

We do not know how or why IBC reduces muscle soreness. Science has not even established the causes of DOMS, although circumstantial evidence implicates microscopic muscle damage and the resulting accumulation of biochemical breakdown products in overworked muscles. We do know that during the elevated heart rate of the IBC workout, the heart pumps more blood at a higher pressure to working muscles, delivering more nutrients and removing metabolic waste products faster. The IBC workout may flush away the causes of muscle soreness before it has a chance to develop, or repair more rapidly the micro-structural muscle damage that results from vigorous exercise.

Whatever the scientific explanation, the reduction of muscle soreness lies at the heart of the integrated exercise revolution. Muscle soreness is widely recognized as one of the most significant barriers to exercise initiation, adherence, and progression, a hurdle for the casual exerciser and the professional athlete alike. Legions of scientists have searched diligently for decades, looking for the magic bullet to banish DOMS. They've tried massage, stretching, cryotherapy, ibuprofen, vitamin E supplements, isoflavones, and even that all-purpose magic potion, fish oil, with no success. The long search is over; the cure for Delayed Onset Muscle Soreness is IBC. You can start and sustain your IBC program, grow fitter faster than any other system we have experienced, get your weight under control quickly—and experience little or no muscle soreness.

The reduction of soreness in IBC is more than a matter of comfort. Delayed Onset Muscle Soreness not only hurts, but also stiffens your muscles, makes them weaker, reduces the range of motion around the joint operated by the sore muscles, changes the way you move, and makes you more prone to injury. IBC's reduction of DOMS opens new vistas. It means that your muscles recover faster from your exercise, which means they can develop faster, imparting greater efficiency to your exercise program.

Freed from DOMS, you can get into better physical shape faster, and reach new heights with less risk of injury, in any given time. Almost everyone has longed for a way to look better fast at one time or another—during the few weeks before your high school reunion, for example, or in the brief spring that precedes your bikini summer. Often getting in the best shape possible in the minimum amount of time is a matter of success or failure—for example, in the limited pre-season of a sports team. Sometimes getting in good physical shape fast can be a matter of life and death—for example, the short conditioning program for emergency workers, first responders, police, and firefighters, or the few short weeks of military boot camp.

The reduction of muscle soreness in IBC has another implication—it means that you can build IBC into your whole life without ever worrying about intolerable pain—or, for that matter, any pain at all—during or between your workouts. Expunging muscle soreness from exercise eliminates a whole suite of negative psychological associations with physical activity, and lies at the heart of the IBC motto: *Less pain, more gain.*

Cardio Is Alive and Well.

IBC bowls over some other sacred cows, too, such as the role of cardiovascular exercise. Professional bodybuilders have long deemphasized cardio (aerobic) exercise, and even discouraged it as a diversion from building muscle. Some weightlifting experts likewise minimize aerobics, or suggest doing it last to avoid draining energy. In their defense, the science of exercise physiology until recently appeared to support this view. A few older studies suggested that combining endurance (cardio) and strength training (weightlifting) reduced the gains of both. Scientists even developed a term for it—the interference effect.

Recent research, however, is dispelling the interference myth, and the scientific results summarized in chapter 3 may put it to rest. The people we trained showed no interference from integrated cardio and resistance training. On the contrary, they showed massive synergisms, or additive effects, between cardio and other forms of exercise. The women we trained in IBC, for example, gained firm muscle mass at twice the rate of the best conventional exercise prescription with no sign of bulking up, and they shed fat at three times the rate without even trying to lose weight. The men showed comparable gains in well-sculpted muscle. The rates of muscle growth we have seen with IBC are higher than any other drug-free training regime. Neither did the athletes we trained using IBC showed any sign of drained energy. On the contrary, the men's soccer team play became electric in intensity. Their opponents could not keep up with them, particularly in the all-important second half (chapter 3).

Some commentators have gone so far as to wonder whether cardio is dead, based on recent slow-motion (anaerobic) exercise systems. Time and research will tell whether slow-motion exercise provides any new benefits. In the meantime, it is biologically certain that unless you elevate your heart rate, you cannot condition all three of your body's energy systems. Training your third gear, your aerobic energy system, occurs only when you elevate your heart rate for prolonged periods. IBC conditions all three of your energy systems (chapter 2), which may be one reason people find IBC so energizing. As long as humans have a heart, cardio is alive and well.

Myth Busting.

IBC lays these and numerous other myths of exercise to rest. We will discuss these myths and puncture them systematically throughout this book, using Myth Busters, one of the motivational tools (chapter 8) that supports IBC. Myth Busters will help you create and sustain a new belief system that is not only more accurate and up to date, based on the most recent scientific understanding, but also more supportive of your IBC program and its continuation for life. You will find the Myth Buster process at work in sidebars throughout this book, like the following one.

Myth Buster 1: No Pain, No Gain

THE MYTH: Exercise hurts too much. I can't handle the pain.

A generation of exercisers has grown up under the misapprehension that exercise is supposed to hurt. It isn't. In an evolutionary sense, good physical condition ensured the survival of our hunter-gatherer ancestors. Why would evolution make something hurt if it is essential for survival? It wouldn't, and it didn't. Pain is generally nature's way of telling us something is amiss, something is wrong inside, and unless we mind it quickly, it could get worse. Pain is a precursor to injury, and injury can end an exercise program or an athletic career.

Exercise pain can take two forms—immediate and residual. Immediate pain can occur during exercise, while residual soreness takes a few hours to arise and lasts for up to several days. Some immediate exercise pain may be unavoidable, depending on the type of exercise you do and your history. If you are older and have led an active life, for example, you may have some past injuries to deal with when you exercise. Mild muscle burn is also unavoidable sometimes, as lactic acid accumulates. Most pain during exercise, however, is unacceptable and avoidable. IBC purposely focuses your attention on any pain signals so you can modify your exercise routine to minimize pain and reduce the risk of injury.

The residual pain of exercise that manifests as muscle soreness and stiffness is Delayed Onset Muscle Soreness, or DOMS. It can start a few hours after conventional high-intensity exercise and persist for up to several days, and it can be debilitating. IBC minimizes this residual pain, too, which means you can exercise as hard as you want without any fear of retribution the next day. Because your muscles recover faster from exercise, you may be able to work out more frequently if that suits your goals.

IBC stabilizes joints, strengthens bones, and conditions ligaments and tendons. It's the best exercise approach to minimize and manage pain both during and between workouts, naturally, and without drugs.

THE REALITY: Nature did not intend exercise to hurt, and when done right, it doesn't. Scratch *No pain, no gain* and replace it with the IBC motto: *Less pain, more gain.*

The IBC Myth Buster

MYTH: Exercise is painful.

FACT: IBC reduces muscle pain and minimizes other pain to maximize gain—and spares far more pain than it causes.

Your Road Map to Integrated Body Conditioning

Now you know how IBC originated, how it works, what it has done for my life, and what it could do for yours. The guiding purpose of this book is to enable you to implement your own IBC program quickly and painlessly. Part 1 lays the foundation, while Part 2 is your performance manual—a step-by-step guide to the beginning, intermediate, and advanced IBC workout. Part 3 shows you how to personalize and customize your IBC workout program and keep it going for life. By the time you have finished reading this book, you will know:

- The underlying rationale for IBC (chapters 2 and 3).
- How to do IBC safely at any level—beginning (chapter 4), intermediate (chapter 5), or advanced (chapter 6).
- How to customize IBC to suit your interests, needs, and goals (chapter 7).
- How to get and stay motivated for exercise (chapter 8).
- What IBC can do for you, regardless of your current status and even if you belong to a clinically defined special population (chapter 9).
- How to make IBC an enduring and integral part of your life (chapter 10).

You will also appreciate the title of this book. We could never have used the term *miracle,* or even written this book, without the confidence that IBC can work wonders for you, too.

Why You Should Do the Miracle Workout

Part 1 of The Miracle Workout *provides the background you need to develop your IBC program. It describes the rationale, principles, and practices of IBC, and highlights the scientific evidence that distinguishes it from other approaches to exercise. Part 1 concludes with the story of the first athletic team to train with IBC and the records it set on its way to the NCAA West Region championship and the NCAA Division III national championship play-offs two years running.*

2

The Art of the Miracle Workout

Before you commit your time and energy to IBC, you deserve the assurance that it is the soundest possible program to create *your* perfect body. Toward this end, this chapter explains the rationale of IBC. We'll look at its principles and practices, see how and why evolution first invented it, and find out why IBC is so effective in conditioning your body system. We will then explore the biological universals of exercise, so you will better appreciate how IBC incorporates them. This will also give you all the tools you need to evaluate any workout program, including the one you may be doing now, and compare it with IBC. It will also set the stage for using your exercise yardstick to evaluate IBC based on science (chapter 3).

The Evolutionary Roots of IBC

Where did integrated exercise come from? The brief answer is evolution. Humans appeared in recognizable form nearly a million years ago, and during all but the last 10,000 years our ancestors were hunter-gatherers, roaming the earth to capture and collect whatever sustenance they could find. The forces of natural selection assembled most of our genetic material during that long hunter-gatherer history. We begin exploring the rationale of IBC by discussing our hominid ancestors—the cave dwellers—for the simple reason that we have their genes. Our common genetic makeup means that whatever physical activity hunter-gatherers did to survive provides the best guidance for contemporary exercise programs.

Based on the activities of the few remaining hunter-gatherer peoples, such as the ¡Kung! Bushmen of Namibia, our cave-dwelling ancestors probably did not exercise at all. Exercise is purposeful physical activity done for its own sake. Early hominids got all the physical activity they needed staying alive from day to day, hunting and gathering, dancing and playing, making war and making love, and handing us the genes for the same activities.

The most striking feature of hunter-gatherer activities is that they were integrated. That is, all body systems participated. The hearts of hunters pounded as they used their brains and muscles to stalk and kill, dismember and carry home their prey. The hearts of gatherers raced as they used their brains to identify and find valuable species, trekked throughout their nomadic lives, flexed and bent to gather nature's harvest, and lifted, hiked, and lugged it back to the clan. In women and men alike, brain and heart, muscle and bone all worked together as a unit.

Evolution prepared the human body to attain peak physical condition when all the cylinders are firing. Our ancestors earned and passed on to us the genes for integrated exercise. The lifestyle of modern industrial society, however, deviates from nature's original design in that food is now abundant, and both work and play are more sedentary. Our bodies respond to nature's deflected intent with the modern maladies—heart disease, obesity, and metabolic syndrome, including diabetes.

We can't turn back the clock and live like hunter-gatherers. It was a hard life, and there are too many people on the planet now anyway. Our hunter-gatherer genes, however, impose a stark choice: exercise or suffer. Our ancestors did not have to exercise, but we do, to compensate for the present-day flood of excess food and dearth of physical activity. We must meet the very different challenges of modern civilization with the genes hunter-gatherers bequeathed us, and that means we need integrated exercise.

Child's Play Is Integrated Exercise

Integrated physical activity characterizes not only our evolution, but also our childhood. If your childhood was like mine, contemporary distractions like televisions and computers didn't exist yet. Even if you had a TV, you probably spent many of your nonschool hours at play. Only in recent years has TV supplanted play as the primary childhood recreation.

Recall the details of just one of those childhood play activities: swinging. You climb onto the seat, lean back, extend your arms and legs, and pull the ropes, and the swing arcs forward and up toward the sky. At its apogee, you contract your abdominal core, flex your arms and legs, push the ropes, and shift your weight forward; the swing arcs back. Soon your heart races as you pull and extend, push and flex. After a few minutes, time stood still, and if you stayed with it long enough you might even have entered the timeless zone of the runner's high. You did not have a term for it then, though. It was just plain fun.

When children swing or wrestle, or ride a bike, or play on monkey bars, their hearts race while they contract and relax their muscles. You'll recognize this as the same integrated physical activity practiced by our cave-dwelling ancestors. As they grow, children increasingly bring other faculties to bear in play. To the joy of swinging, we add progressively more mindful games—hide-and-seek, kick the can, and then team games and sports that require ever-greater strategic thinking. This natural progression engages the brain in stages, as mind and body learn to work together and with other people. Maybe play is nature's way of preparing us for the integrated exercise of the hunter-gatherer adulthood, as programmed in our genes. IBC incorporates the same principles, and that may be why people who do the workout often say it feels like play.

The modern lifestyle not only confounded evolution's intent for adulthood, but also derailed evolution's expectations for childhood. We start school nearly as soon as we can talk, and quickly learn to stifle internal impulses for physical activity and sit quietly, or face the consequences. When children rebel against such unnatural constraints, we label them with complex diagnoses and medicate them. When the school bell rings at the end of the day, contemporary children are likely to switch on the television, turn to video games, or surf the Internet. It is little wonder that the most recent childhood epidemics are obesity and depression.

For modern children and adults alike, the need to exercise independently from play, education, and work is new, from an evolutionary standpoint. Exercise as a stand-alone, purposeful activity is an artifact of compartmentalized modern life. Given our genetics, however, we ignore exercise at our peril.

Condition the Body System

Our ancestors knew, and contemporary indigenous peoples still practice, something many of us have forgotten: Everything is connected to everything else, on large scales and small, in ecosystems and the human body. This holistic perspective has reemerged in modern society in many ways, but none more surprising than within the innards of electronic devices. Complex systems such as computers, for example, emerge from individual parts—resistors, capacitors, silicon chips.

Their proper function, however, depends on the interactions among those parts, and the language of those interactions is systems theory. Electronic engineers and mathematicians developed systems theory in the middle of the 20th century. It immediately fertilized existing disciplines such as the neurosciences and psychology, and spawned new fields like ecology.

Systems theory provides invaluable insight for exercise, too. Consider a sports team, for example, as a system composed of the players, which are its parts. The success of a team depends on the players themselves, but more fundamentally on their interactions during competition. Championship teams are often those with the strongest players, but always those that operate most effectively as a single, interacting system. Conversely, the best players don't necessarily make the best team. At the 2004 Summer Olympics in Athens, the U.S. men's basketball Dream Team arguably had the best players, but their team play was less developed, enabling other teams to sometimes prevail.

The human body is also a collection of interdependent parts, or organs, each providing a reciprocated benefit to every other. The heart pumps blood to the kidneys, and the kidneys purify blood for the heart. Muscles create movement, which brings food to the stomach and intestines, which prepare nutrients for the muscles, and so on across the whole system. Optimum body function depends on the capacity of the individual parts, but it is the quality of their interactions that defines health and wellness, physical fitness, and peak performance. The interaction of the parts determines the action of the whole, and what is good for the whole is best for the parts.

Conditioning the human body invites the same systems approach as coaching a team or designing a computer. Instead of focusing on any single body part, optimum physical conditioning trains the entire, interacting system. This is the central rationale for IBC. Any exercise program that tries to condition individual parts without attention to the whole can't work as well. Systems theory rules whether the whole is a radio, the brain, an ecosystem, a sports team, or the human body.

If your exercise goals include great guns, for example—bodybuilder lingo for well-developed biceps—the conventional exercise prescription is to do plenty of heavy arm curls, with rest between each set of repetitions. IBC, in contrast, approaches the human body as an interactive system. If it's bulging biceps you seek, or washboard abs, or tight glutes, don't limit your attention to these individual targets as if they existed in a vacuum. Train the whole system instead. Your biceps, belly, or derriere will know the difference, and each will develop to its maximum genetic potential.

FIGURE 2.1
SEVEN PRINCIPLES OF INTEGRATED BODY CONDITIONING

IBC encompasses seven broad principles. Apply them and you are on your way to the best body you can have:

1. Integrated exercise. Include cardiovascular, resistance, and Range of Motion (ROM, or flexibility) exercise in every workout.

2. Cardio-driving. Work out at a properly elevated heart rate, determined by your starting level and your exercise goals, by cardio-accelerating before other exercises.

3. Body consciousness. Use biofeedback to listen to your body when you work out.

4. Progression. Achieve steady growth, using perceived exertion and perceived pain to govern your rate of progression.

5. Minimize pain. Monitor and manage pain, with the purpose of minimizing it and avoiding injury, to maximize gain.

6. Balance. Condition the whole body system, with balance across muscles, joints, the three energy systems, the year, and your life.

7. Mind-body connection. Your mind and your body are a single, indivisible system that you use to maximize exercise results.

Seven Principles of IBC

Systems theory provides the basis for seven guiding principles of IBC (figure 2.1). Most of these principles are not new, but IBC puts them together purposefully for the first time. You already know the first principle: Do integrated exercise. That means you incorporate the three major exercise modes—cardio, resistance, flexibility—into every workout. You also know the second principle—cardio-driving. Cardio-accelerate, or elevate your heart rate, into your training window and then do other kinds of exercise. Elevating your heart rate increases your core body temperature as much as 5 degrees Fahrenheit, accelerating the biochemical reactions that underlie muscle contraction. Cardio-driving also triggers the release by the brain of natural opiate-like substances, endorphins and enkephalons, which may underlie the runner's high. Above all, cardio-driving force-feeds and speed-cleans your muscles, so they work better and grow faster with less soreness.

The third principle of IBC is body consciousness. IBC invites you to listen to your body continuously while you exercise. You monitor your heart rate during IBC to stay in your training window, optimize physical exertion levels, and minimize pain signals. Body consciousness is the basis of IBC's method of progression, which is one reason it enables such rapid development.

Progression is the fourth principle of IBC. You strive constantly to improve by increasing your exercise workload. A centerpiece of IBC is the method of progression. You monitor your perceived pain and exertion using a well-established scale, and progress from one workout to the next on that basis. You will find progression in IBC easy, for three reasons. First, you grow stronger with each IBC workout. What was hard yesterday becomes easy tomorrow. Second, you always progress at your own pace, determined by your perceived levels of exertion and pain. Third, once you reach a certain level of health, fitness, or performance, defined by your exercise goals, you switch into maintenance mode. Maintenance takes less effort, entails variety, and does not demand constant progression.

The fifth principle of IBC is to minimize pain. Pain is an ally because it warns of impending injury, which slows growth. Even a minor injury can set a workout program back weeks or months. If you are an athlete, it can end a season or a career. The stronger and fitter you get, however, the less likely you are to be injured. IBC uses the strategy of monitoring any pain to make sure it never exceeds what you would consider weak. We will give you the tools for that shortly.

The sixth principle of IBC is balance—not the kind that keeps you upright, although that improves dramatically with exercise. Balance here means that whenever you exercise one muscle, such as the biceps, you also exercise its antagonist, the triceps, ensuring symmetrical strength and stabilized joints. Research on professional hockey players shows that balanced strength training protects against injury. Unbalanced exercise creates asymmetrical strength that distorts joints, as illustrated by a study published in the June 2003 *Annals of Internal Medicine*. For many years, doctors advised people with arthritic knees to exercise the large muscles in the front upper thigh, the quadriceps, by doing leg extensions. The *Annals* article reported that this prescription worsened knee arthritis in 230 arthritis patients followed over 18 months. Unbalanced exercise is counterproductive whether arthritis is involved or not.

Balance also means strengthening all the primary and secondary joints of the body, so each part can assist every other to grow and develop as fast and as far as your genetics allow. IBC balances exercise type across cardiovascular, stretching, and resistance exercise, ensuring reciprocal strengthening of your whole body system, including your three energy systems. IBC incorporates balance across seasons (cross-training, periodization), keeping you challenged and interested. Balance across life means eating and sleeping well (chapter 10), which interacts reciprocally with integrated exercise.

The seventh principle of IBC is the mind–body connection. The mind–body connection is a corollary of systems theory, which regards the mind and body as a single, interacting entity. Because they are one, the functions of mind and body are inseparable. Eastern traditions long ago understood and worked with the mind–body connection, applying it to physical conditioning in Yoga, Tai Chi, and the martial arts. IBC borrows from this ancient tradition.

An implication of the mind–body connection is that you maximize the mentation process when you're physically fit. A recent study on pre-adolescent boys found that fit subjects showed greater heart rate reactivity to a mentally challenging task than their unfit counterparts, suggesting that a fit body supports mental activity better. Mental acuity during aging also remains highest when people stay in physical condition. Dr. Joseph Mercola writes:

> *Exercise is a very potent way to ward off Alzheimer's. Previous research showed the odds of developing Alzheimer's were nearly quadrupled in people who were less active during their leisure time, between the ages of 20 and 60, compared with their peers.*[1]

Physical conditioning affects other functions of the brain, including emotion and mood. Any exercise, particularly vigorous exercise, reduces depression. Similarly, an acute bout of exercise reduces anxiety dramatically, even when the intensity of the exercise is low or moderate. And if you are like many people, IBC at intermediate and particularly advanced levels is a guaranteed ticket into the territory of the runner's high—or simply, the zone.

IBC Harnesses the Zone

In her book *Ultimate Fitness,* Gina Kolata interviewed people who experience the runner's high regularly. One called it "an extracorporeal experience" and added, "it is exercise in a particular way when everything is working and I'm in shape and just flying."[2] Another noted, "it has that well-being kind of feeling, that Superman . . . Feeling."[3] Yet another put it this way: "You worked so hard to get out of the earth's gravity and now it's so beautiful. You're floating."[4] Some exercisers mentioned the feeling that comes following a workout: "I still feel ecstatic for a half hour or more . . . something seems to have changed in my brain."[5] No one knows what that *something* is, but natural chemicals released within the brain—endorphins and enkephalons—may play a role. These are first detectable in cerebrospinal fluid 20 minutes into a hard run, right about when the feeling of the runner's high starts.

Conventional exercise programs consider time in the zone as a side effect of vigorous exercise, a kind of bonus prize that rewards hard work. IBC, in contrast, harnesses the runner's high to a higher purpose. Instead of an incidental treat, time in the zone is a systematic tool by which you accelerate your development. IBC achieves this aim by juxtaposing exercise that sustains the runner's high—aerobics—with other exercises that normally do not—ROM and resistance exercise. IBC therefore focuses the power of the zone on the development of body flexibility, muscle strength, and muscle endurance.

The Three-Step IBC Program

IBC puts diverse forms of exercise together in the same workout. At the end point, you integrate cardio with stretching and with resistance exercise. You get there in three simple steps, or stages, as in the analogy of the three-section musical band (chapter 1). In the first step, the cardio phase, you do aerobic exercise alone, until you are in adequate cardio shape—that is, until you reach specific milestones demonstrating that your heart is in condition for the second step. This takes a week to a month, depending on your initial physical condition and goals. You will then be ready to cardio-drive your body system safely and comfortably to its full potential.

The second step, the cardiorom phase, adds bending and stretching exercises (flexibility training) to develop full range of motion around every joint. Strength training sometimes neglects ROM exercise, which is a mistake. Your muscles have to work through a full natural range to reach their full potential strength. The cardiorom phase integrates ROM exercise with cardio by alternating bouts of aerobic exercise with bending and stretching exercises. It will take anywhere from a week or two to a month, depending on your physical condition and goals.

Then, when you are ready, take the third step to the fully integrated cardiolift phase. This is the final, fully integrated IBC workout. Here you add resistance training—weightlifting—to your routine by alternating resistance exercises with brief bouts of cardio-accelerating aerobic exercise. At the end of each cardiolift workout, you do ROM exercises to cool down, completing the circle.

That's how IBC incorporates three traditionally distinct approaches to exercise—aerobics, flexibility or ROM exercises, and resistance training or weightlifting—into a single, seamless exercise system, incorporating them all into one efficient and comprehensive workout. That is when something new happens, something you may not have felt since you were a child—or, for that matter, ever. All three sections of your body's band finally play together as a single instrument.

The Practices of IBC

Chapters 4–6 detail IBC practices at the beginning, intermediate, and advanced levels. A general orientation now will help you understand the process and advantages of IBC before doing the workouts. IBC builds your body in steps that begin with cardio and then integrate ROM and resistance exercises. You condition your cardiovascular system because your heart supports integrated exercise. Cardiovascular exercise is not in itself integrated—it trains mainly your aerobic metabolism (*long-term energy system training*) and whatever muscles you use to cardio-drive. That is an adequate end goal of some exercisers, such as joggers, runners, and cyclists. Though limited, cardio exercise is the best way to strengthen your cardiopulmonary system (*aerobic capacity*), which is the most important single contributor to general health and wellness and the best single indicator of longevity.

To launch the first cardio phase of an IBC workout, you may want to review a pertinent Myth Buster to reinforce your motivation. Then choose your favorite cardiovascular exercise, and start slow and easy at your own pace. Gradually increase your cardio workout intensity in successive workouts until you can stay in your identified cardio training heart rate window for 20 or 30 minutes comfortably—with a perceived exertion of *strong* or less, and a perceived pain of *weak* or less. (These rating scales are detailed in chapters 4–6.) The most obvious quantitative indicator of increased cardiovascular strength is the steady reduction in your average heart rate at any given exercise's intensity and duration. (We'll show you how to monitor that later.) You will delight in the progress you make, which is often noticeable from one workout to the next.

When your heart is ready, launch the second step in your IBC program, cardiorom, by integrating ROM with cardio exercise. Just stretch and bend (*body flexibility*) while your heart rate is elevated. Select a good basic sequence of flexibility exercises, or use those shown in chapters 4–6, to target all your body joints: hips and shoulders (the primary joints), knees and elbows (secondary), and wrists and ankles (tertiary). Warm up, cardio-accelerate, and then do your first ROM exercise while your heart rate is still elevated well into your cardiovascular conditioning window, which we'll define in chapters 4–6.

In your very first cardiorom workout, you will feel a new kind of flexibility. The elevated heart rate and body temperature created by cardio exercise will seem to fluidize your body and minimize the mild discomfort that some people feel when they stretch and bend. ROM exercises generally require less physical effort than the initial warm-up and intermittent cardio exercise, however, so when you do a ROM exercise your heart rate will drop out of your training window. A brief (one-minute) cardio-acceleration bout will elevate it for your second ROM exercise. After that exercise, do another cardio-acceleration, your third ROM exercise, and so on to the end of your ROM sequence. Cardiorom is therefore a comprehensive stretch-and-bend workout done at an elevated heart rate.

Soon you are ready to move to the third step of IBC, by integrating cardio exercise with resistance training—contracting and relaxing your muscles against an external load. The most familiar example of resistance exercise is weightlifting, which is why we call this stage of IBC the cardiolift phase. Resistance training is essential to muscle development (*muscle strength, muscle endurance*), and builds strong cartilage and ligaments, bones and joints. The comparatively explosive movements of resistance training also condition your phosphorous energy system (*short-term energy system training*) and engage your anaerobic energy system (*medium-term energy system training*).

There are at least two other major benefits of resistance training that you can't get any other way. First, resistance exercise induces long-term repair of deliberately stressed muscle tissue by firing up your body's repair metabolism (catabolism). Second, resistance exercise stimulates your body to grow new muscle (anabolism), which burns yet more calories. Resistance training therefore creates muscle while it melts fat (*body composition*), and is the best way to achieve and maintain a desirable weight without calorie-restricting diets. Resistance exercise combined with proper diet is also the best and only natural antidote for osteoporosis (porous bone disease), an affliction that is fast approaching epidemic proportions and strikes women the hardest.

Start your fully integrated cardiolift workout with a warm-up to raise your heart rate into your cardiovascular training window. Then move directly to your first weightlifting exercise, following the pattern of the cardiorom phase. Alternate resistance exercises with brief cardio-acceleration bouts that keep your heart rate in your training window. Select your resistance exercises (chapters 4–6) to achieve overall balance across your main body joints and the whole body, including the all-important core—the abdomen and lower back. A balanced workout requires ROM exercise, so finish your cardiolift workout with a ROM session.

The three steps to the fully integrated IBC workout—cardio, cardiorom, cardiolift—are extremely simple in practice. Deconditioned college students who have never before exercised learn the beginning IBC workout in a single session, after which it is second nature. Even the advanced IBC workout takes college athletes only a couple of sessions to master. Most important, the same deconditioned college students strongly preferred IBC to the six other workouts we tested (chapter 3). IBC is more enjoyable (*the fun factor*).

As we've seen (chapter 1), a key element to the rapid development made possible through IBC is its method of progression—the way you increase your workload from one workout to the next. Exercisers sometimes leave progression to chance or mood—*how I feel today* determines how hard to work. A laissez-faire approach to an exercise workload is fine and even appropriate, sometimes, but if you want to develop to higher levels, it is unhelpful for one simple reason: adaptation. As you progress in IBC, you grow stronger and fitter so fast that your body adapts to any given workload. You may already have experienced adaptation. When you start a garden, for example, it can be hard work, but by harvesttime you have become accustomed to it and it feels easier.

The same is true for any exercise program—what was heavy yesterday is light tomorrow. Unless you continuously add to your workload, your muscles are no longer stimulated, and they stop getting stronger. In exercise, you progress or stagnate. The IBC method of progression is the antidote to adaptation. You progress in each exercise, and from one workout to the next, automatically at your own pace, by optimizing your perceived exertion and minimizing your perceived pain using a simple and well-known rating scale. You then decide to stay where you are or progress immediately upon completing each exercise. When you start your next IBC workout, you know exactly what you have to do because your body told you during your last workout.

As long as you are healthy and injury-free, the IBC method of progression empowers you to advance steadily for months at a time without stagnating, or plateauing. The IBC method of auto-progression will carry you to heights of fitness, strength, and endurance that you might never have reached otherwise. It also melts body fat and creates new layers of muscle up to three times faster than the best conventional exercise prescription. IBC's unique method of progression is easy to apply in practice, and is one of the three elements of IBC that enables accelerated development.

Your Exercise Yardstick

Every human body works on the same universal biological principles, and an exercise program that addresses all of them is the best choice for anyone. These exercise universals are the biological common denominators of exercise; they form the

FIGURE 2.2
THE SEVEN DIMENSIONS OF EXERCISE

There are seven dimensions to any form of exercise. Use these dimensions as metrics by which you can evaluate your exercise program and compare it with IBC:

1. Muscle strength—how much weight you can lift, pull, or push. It's measured by the one-repetition maximum, or 1-RM, for the corresponding exercise.

2. Muscle endurance—how many times you can repeat a lift, push, or pull, using as the resistance either your body weight (as in push-ups) or 50–65 percent of your 1-RM (in exercises that use dumbbells, barbells, or machines).

3. Aerobic capacity—how much oxygen your body uses at peak exertion, measured as your VO_{2max} (milliliters of oxygen you consume per kilogram of body weight per minute). It's the gold standard of physical fitness.

4. Body flexibility—how much of the full range of motion around each joint you can move. The more flexible your body, the greater range of motion you enjoy, and the more muscle strength you can develop.

5. Body composition—what percentage of your body is fat-free mass (mainly muscle and bone) and what percentage is fat. Healthy fat percentages typically range 10–25 percent (toward the lower end for men, the higher for women).

6. Energy systems training. This is addressed, indirectly, by training the above five dimensions, which condition all three energy systems—short-term phosphorus, medium-term anaerobic, and long-term aerobic.

7. Fun. The more fun your exercise program is, the more likely you'll be to get started in the first place and then stay with it for life.

basis of an exercise yardstick that you can use to evaluate any exercise program. We'll first construct your yardstick, and then use it to see how any exercise program, including IBC, measures up.

Your exercise yardstick has seven metrics, corresponding to the seven universal dimensions of exercise (figure 2.2). The first five dimensions are muscle strength, muscle endurance, aerobic capacity, body flexibility, and body composition (the proportion of fat-free mass). The sixth cuts across these first five—it is your body's three energy systems (short-term, medium-term, and long-term energy system conditioning). The seventh is how much you enjoy your exercise program—the fun factor.

The first of these universal dimensions of exercise, muscle strength, refers to the most weight you can move a specified distance with a particular muscle group. It is measured by your one-repetition maximum weight, or 1-RM, which establishes the strength of the corresponding muscle or muscles in terms that are easy to understand and assess—how many pounds you can lift, push, or pull. Muscle strength influences strongly how you look and feel. For women, muscle strength translates into a firm, toned look. Contrary to common belief, strength training will not make women get bulky; testosterone, the male hormone, is what produces muscle bulk. For men, muscle strength is therefore associated typically with larger, more sculpted muscles. In addition to looking fit, strength training confers greater bone mineral density and strength, and corresponding protection from injury; increased mobility, which makes life safer and more fun; increased ease of weight control because of more muscle; and that top-of-the-world feeling of full body power, which translates to every moment of everyday life.

Muscle endurance is a measure of how long your muscles can work at any specified load. The standard measure is the number of repetitions you can do without pause of a particular exercise, such as push-ups. The weight you move during push-ups, and many other exercises, is your body weight. If you measure endurance using free weights or machines, the standard weight used to assess endurance is 50–65 percent of your 1-RM for that particular exercise—toward the lower end for women, higher for men. Muscle endurance training imparts that lean, toned, and defined look, accompanied by a feeling of energy, and transfers into everyday life and athletics. When you train for muscle endurance, you feel so energetic that everyday physical activities become a breeze. If you are a senior, you will feel as if you've discovered the fountain of youth, and in a sense you have. Muscle endurance is central to sports such as cycling, soccer, basketball, and swimming.

Aerobic capacity is the third dimension of exercise, and the third metric on the exercise yardstick. The gold standard of physical fitness, aerobic capacity is the maximum oxygen your body can use per unit of body weight in one minute of peak exertion. It is quantified by the VO_{2max}. The higher your VO_{2max}, the greater your aerobic capacity and the better your physical condition. Values of VO_{2max} range from as low as 15 or 20 for healthy, deconditioned adults, to as high as 80 or more for world-class athletes such as six-time Tour de France champion Lance Armstrong. Elite, national-caliber endurance athletes typically have a VO_{2max} value of

50–70. Exercise that develops aerobic capacity includes any endurance activity or sport, including running on a treadmill, long-distance running, basketball, cross-country skiing, and cycling.

The fourth universal register on your exercise yardstick is body flexibility, technically called Range of Motion or ROM. Body flexibility is what gives you that delicious feeling of supple pliancy that most of us had as children, which often fades as we grow older. Increased flexibility is important for pain management, particularly as we age. Lower back pain, which afflicts 70 percent of Americans at some point in their lives, is associated with lack of flexibility in the trunk and hamstrings (the back of the thigh). Greater flexibility reduces overuse injuries by half, and it's associated with reduced muscle soreness and lower incidence of muscle injury in athletes. Flexibility training is also crucial to strength development. College students who combined ROM training with weight training got 33 percent stronger in a 10-week workout period, compared with a 10 percent gain for people who lifted weights alone. You can't develop full strength or endurance around any joint in your body unless you can operate that joint through its full range of motion.

A well-publicized recent review of the scientific literature on stretching found no conclusive evidence that stretching before exercise prevents injury. It's true that stretching before or instead of a warm-up is neither necessary nor beneficial, and can be harmful. Stretching after you warm up, however, confers benefits that range from fewer lower back and muscle problems to increased strength. If you suffer limited range of motion around any joint—say, from an old injury—flexibility training after a thorough warm-up is especially important.

Body composition is the fifth dimension of exercise. It's defined by your body's ratio of fat-free mass (muscle and bone) to adipose tissue (fat). Typical healthy fat percentages in the human body range 5–25 percent. A body composition of 5 percent fat is getting dangerously low for women and most men, but sometimes occurs in elite athletes such as marathon runners. At the other extreme, 25 percent fat is the threshold for being overweight by one definition. A healthy intermediate value is 10–20 percent—a little lower in this range for males, and a little higher for females.

A variety of laboratory techniques measure body composition, but the most practical is the skinfold test. Half of body fat is subcutaneous—it lies just beneath the skin. A trained person can measure skinfold thickness at specific body sites and plug the numbers into standard equations to determine body composition within a few percentage points. You can also do the jiggle test, which is approximate and easy. On your tiptoes stand naked in front of a mirror, and drop your heels suddenly to the floor. If you neither see nor feel any jiggle, you're probably in the lower

Myth Buster 2: Starvation Dieting

THE MYTH: Calorie-reduction diets are the best way to lose weight.

The latest bestsellers on diet pack bookstore shelves—the Atkins diet, the South Beach diet, and so on. There's a big market—two-thirds of Americans are overweight, and one-third are "obese," meaning their body fat makes up 25 percent or more of their weight. The U.S. Centers for Disease Control (CDC) has warned repeatedly that we are getting too fat and dying from the diseases of obesity—heart disease, diabetes, and high blood pressure. The CDC released a report in 2003 stating that one in three Americans born in 2000 will develop diabetes unless we change exercise and diet habits. Obesity has even overtaken smoking as the leading preventable cause of premature death.

The global picture is no rosier. The United Nations World Health Organization (WHO) reports that health problems related to improper diet and exercise are a leading cause of global death and disability, killing 56.5 million people every year. That's half as many people every year as died in *all* armed conflicts during the 20th century. The WHO is developing minimum standards for diet and exercise to address this national and global epidemic.

Unfortunately, the severity of the obesity epidemic has helped cloak all kinds of fad diets in science. We are particularly afflicted with the myth that the best way to lose weight is calorie-reduction diets. That is true for some special populations (chapter 9), or if you are consuming far more calories than you are burning. Such diets also slow the metabolism, however, and reduce the calories we burn. The irony is that in order to lose weight, we starve—which actually impedes weight loss.

The best and only lasting way to shed fat and keep it off is to incorporate exercise into your life, combined as necessary with calorie consciousness. IBC dramatically increases lean body mass, and at the same time conditions your energy systems; both of these actions burn even more calories. If you exercise regularly and eat a balanced diet, your body seeks and maintains its natural equilibrium weight. IBC will shed pounds far more effectively than calorie-reduction diets, and bring you to your ideal weight automatically.

THE REALITY: Calorie-reduction dieting, while appropriate in some cases, can work against weight loss; exercise is an essential step to a healthy body composition.

The IBC Myth Buster

MYTH: Dieting is the best way to lose fat.

FACT: IBC is the ideal foundation for a comprehensive weight loss and maintenance program.

range of percent body fat (5–15 percent); if you see or feel some jiggle, you're likely in the middle range (15–25 percent); and if you see or feel a whole lot of jiggle, you're probably in the upper range (25 percent and up).

For several generations now, we've learned an erroneous way to achieve a healthy body composition—starvation dieting. Recall that your genes are those of a hunter-gatherer, and they evolved at a time when food supply depended on a variable environment. When you reduce caloric intake much below your daily expenditure for any length of time, your body responds as if food is scarce, and your metabolism slows to conserve fat. That's evolution's way of keeping the hunter-gatherer alive through hard times. Conserving fat is probably not exactly what you had in mind by dieting, but that is what your hunter-gatherer genes decree (see the sidebar).

Nature provides two ways to increase the amount of calories we burn—eating and exercising. Burning calories by eating may seem too good to be true. Every time you have even a small meal, however, your body's digestive response turns up your metabolism by as much as 25 percent for as long as an hour. This thermic response burns extra calories, which is one reason many nutrition experts advise eating many small meals rather than a few big meals each day. Several meals a day can also keep you from getting too hungry and overeating.

The second and more effective way to stoke your calorie furnace is to exercise regularly. You burn some calories during workouts; more important, however, exercise empowers you to burn more calories between workouts. Muscle uses more calories than fat, so the greater muscle mass you create, the more calories you will burn even at rest, every moment of every day and night, even while you're sleeping. Exercise also conditions your three energy systems, which keeps them burning calories at an accelerated rate day and night. Unless you belong to a special clinical population (chapter 9), you can control your weight best by eating a healthy, balanced diet—the integrated diet (chapter 10)—and revving up your metabolism with IBC. Your body will seek its natural weight automatically, and possibly spare you the need for calorie-reduction diets.

If you do belong to a special clinical population, particularly the obese (chapter 9), combine IBC with calorie limitation, or at least become calorie conscious. If you are overweight, you cannot ignore your diet—even if you are not technically obese. Many studies show that a combination of diet and exercise is the best way to shed pounds and keep them off permanently. If your goal is to reduce body weight, make sure your diet is healthy (chapter 10), and continue that diet while you implement your IBC program. Your body weight will settle to a lower equilibrium value that reflects a balance of calorie intake and the increased calorie expenditure.

If that equilibrium weight is still greater than you want, you can resort to restricting calorie intake.

That brings us to the sixth metric on the exercise yardstick, energy systems training. It's the most misunderstood and underrated aspect of exercise, but the basics are straightforward. Your body is powered by three discrete but interconnected biochemical pathways, analogous to three gears in a car's standard transmission—short-term energy (first gear), medium-term (second gear), and long-term (third gear). Your short-term energy system is based on phosphorus-containing compounds that break apart to release the energy that powers every movement you make for a period of time lasting from the first few seconds to as long as a minute. This system delivers energy without oxygen, but it depletes quickly and needs replenishment from the next two energy systems.

Your medium-term energy system is also anaerobic—that is, it works without oxygen. You shift in to this second gear during the first 30 seconds of exercise and stay there for the next few minutes. This second gear runs down rapidly, too, however, in part because it produces lactic acid as a by-product, which builds up quickly in your muscles to create that burning sensation that can stop you in your tracks. When your body peaks out in second gear, lactic acid starts to accumulate in your blood. The heart rate at which this accumulation begins in earnest is your lactate threshold. Cross the threshold, and your minutes of exercise at that intensity are numbered. Endurance athletes such as marathon runners and cyclists therefore train to increase their heart rate's lactate threshold, and then compete just beneath it.

The long-term energy system, your body's third gear, is the familiar aerobic system that you condition when you do cardiovascular exercise. Just like your car, your body shifts into third gear at high speeds and for the long haul. The aerobic energy system burns oxygen, kicks in after a few minutes of vigorous exercise, and provides staying power. Endurance athletes rely on the aerobic system because of its ability to sustain intense exercise for long periods without running down. Your aerobic system ultimately replenishes the energy used by your phosphorus and anaerobic systems.

Training all three of your energy systems is crucial, yet often overlooked in exercise prescriptions. You don't have to be a performance athlete to benefit from energy systems training. Your car needs all three gears to transport you even short distances, as in everyday journeys like trips to the grocery store. Similarly, your body needs all three energy systems to power the simplest movements—and to burn every calorie you consume. In practice, and unlike the gears of an automobile, your body's three energy systems overlap during exercise in a kind of biological synchromesh. Training all three energy systems imparts the broadest exercise capacity and confers one of the greatest treasures of IBC—the feeling of boundless energy.

IBC purposely trains all three gears in the same workout. It targets your short-term energy system using brief bursts of all-out exercise, including resistance training (weightlifting, cardio-acceleration). It conditions your medium-term energy system through resistance training and alternating cardio-acceleration bouts. IBC trains your long-term energy system by sustained medium-to-high-intensity cardiovascular exercise. No other exercise system purposely trains all three systems in the same workout. Circuit training comes closest, but it generally emphasizes endurance rather than strength.

The seventh dimension of exercise, fun, is the easiest to understand and, arguably, the most important. If you don't enjoy the process of exercise, you are less likely to reach your destination, whether it's health and wellness, physical fitness, or peak athletic performance. "People become fit through programs that fit them."[6] In applying your exercise yardstick, pay the keenest attention to how much you enjoy whatever system you select. Irrespective of other features, the best exercise program is the one you enjoy the most, and which you will therefore do for life. As you will see shortly (chapter 3), IBC shines when it comes to fun.

Measure Up!

Your exercise yardstick is complete. It has seven metrics, representing the universal dimensions of exercise shown in figure 2.2. If you are already exercising, evaluate your current program using the seven-point yardstick, giving one point for each exercise dimension represented in your exercise program. Most programs score from two to four points on the seven-point scale. That need not be a problem if your program meets your personal exercise goals and if you enjoy it enough to stay with it for the long term.

One exercise program, however, scores seven points; it is the most fun, the most efficient, and therefore takes the least time to achieve any given training result. Prove this for yourself. Go back to the section above titled The Practices of IBC and apply your exercise yardstick. We've made your search easy by enclosing each of the dimensions of exercise that is represented in IBC in italicized print and in parentheses, immediately after the IBC practice that first addresses it. IBC scores a perfect seven, excelling by this measure because it purposely addresses every aspect of conditioning all of your body systems in a single, comprehensive workout that is as easy—or as hard—as you want.

IBC not only measures up to any conventional exercise metric, but is also one of the few exercise programs evaluated by controlled random and double-blind scientific research, to which we now turn. We'll use the exercise yardstick to show how IBC stands head and shoulders above the best conventional exercise prescription. You will also see how IBC brought the UCSC women's soccer team to a new level, and how it helped propel the UCSC men's soccer team to the NCAA West Regional championship and national play-offs two years running.

■ ■ ■

3

The Science of the Miracle Workout

Novel exercise systems or programs appear almost daily on television and in popular fitness magazines, with the vast majority supported mainly by personal testimony. Such new programs generally lack objective, independent, long-term scientific evaluation. How do you know which to believe, and why? IBC is also a new approach to exercise, and merits the same critical evaluation as any exercise program before you commit your time and energy. That's one purpose of the exercise yardstick we constructed in the last chapter. In this chapter, we apply the yardstick to IBC, and to the best conventional exercise prescription, using all the tools that science can muster, to show that IBC enables:

- Three times the fat loss.
- Twice the muscle gain.
- More than double the gain in flexibility.
- Two-thirds greater increase in aerobic capacity.
- Half again the benefit of lowered blood pressure.
- An equal to one-third greater increase in muscle strength.
- An equal to nearly twice the increase in muscle endurance.
- Faster cardiovascular conditioning.
- One-tenth the discomfort from Delayed Onset Muscle Soreness (DOMS).

We will also illustrate the applied results of IBC with the story of the UCSC men's soccer team. These players were unranked before training with IBC but, afterward, moved up in to fifth and then second place in the United States, setting numerous individual and school records along the way.

The Scientific Evidence for IBC

My colleagues in these studies, and some of the student-athletes we had the privilege to train, appear in the photos on following pages. Our research employed five types of scientific evidence to evaluate IBC:

1. Controlled, double-blind, and randomized scientific experiments on selected groups of people who did either IBC or the best conventional exercise program.
2. Survey data, in which a different group rated IBC and compared it with other exercise approaches they had learned.
3. Case studies, in which quantitative data were collected from individuals who have trained with IBC.
4. Testimonial evidence from individuals who have used IBC.
5. Team performance data from the championship USCS men's soccer team before and after training in IBC.

We will highlight the results here. Details, including annotated graphical comparisons using every metric on the exercise yardstick, are published at www. MiracleWorkout.com. Click on "Results," and then on the same headings that appear in this chapter.

Muscle Strength

A Case Study.
I replicated my original self-experiments with the IBC workout on several occasions. In each case, I recorded my workout data using the workout logs described in chapter 6. In one of these replications (winter 2003), my total workload* increased from 10,000 pounds to more than 50,000 in three months. That's a gain in muscle strength of 15 percent per week as measured by total workload, in con-

---

* Total workload is the sum across all exercises in the advanced IBC workout of poundage times the number of sets times the number of repetitions, and provides an indicator of net exercise "volume" over time.

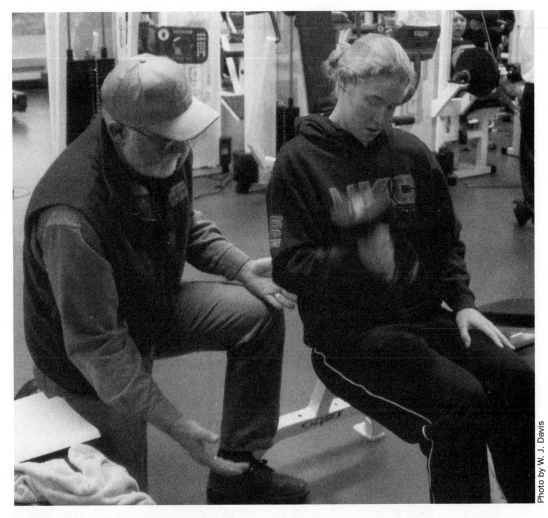

Dr. Dan Wood trains Skye Vendt-Pearce, a member of the women's soccer team, in the seated dumbbell curl.

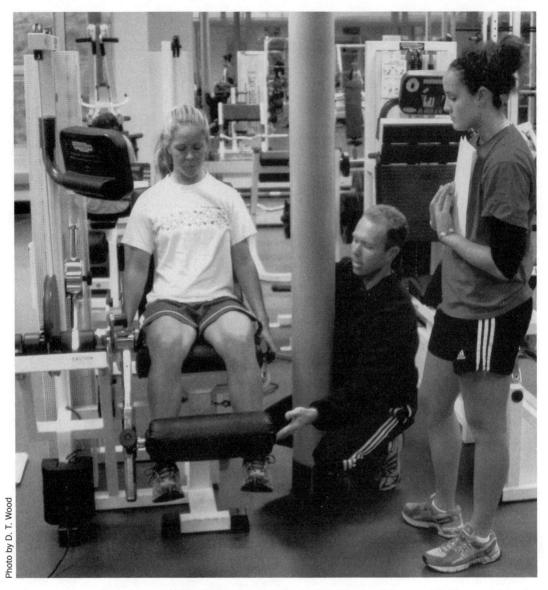

Photo by D. T. Wood

Ryan Andrews trains soccer player Gabriel Craig on the leg extension machine while teammate Courtney Frick observes.

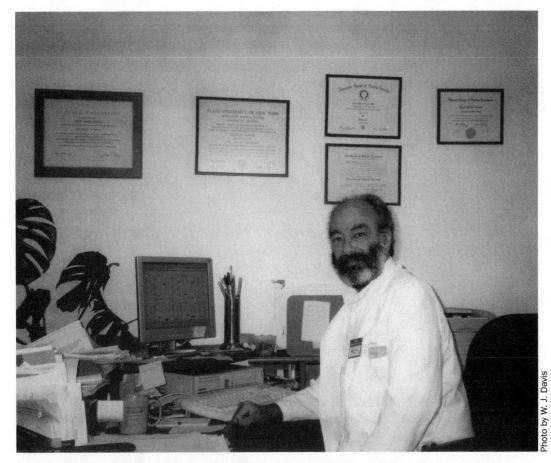

Dr. Les Elkind in his office at the university's Student Health Center, which he directs.

trast to the 3–5 percent per week of the best conventional training programs. I experienced no workload plateau, no Delayed Onset Muscle Soreness, and very little pain from other sources during this 12-week program. In other, similar experiments, I experienced steady growth in muscle strength from the beginning to the end of a six-month gym-based IBC workout, with no plateau in overall workload. Over a lifetime of exercise, I have never found a faster way to grow muscle strength.

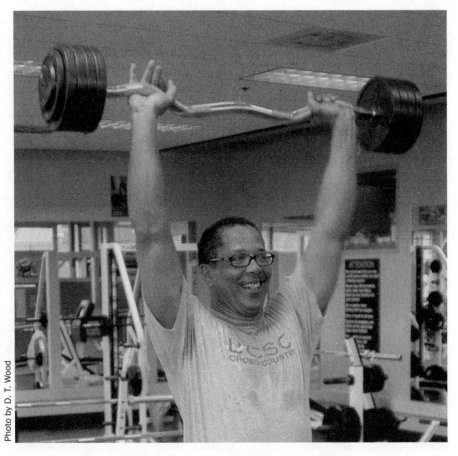

Photo by D. T. Wood

The university's athletic director, Greg Harshaw, stays athletic.

The University of California Experiments*

Case studies are fine, but no match for controlled, randomized, and double-blind scientific experiments such as those we have done with volunteer student-athletes at UCSC. We did two separate experiments in successive years, one with 32 women, the other with 22 men. In both experiments, we compared IBC (the experimental group in each case) with the best conventional exercise prescription (the control group),

---

* All subjects in these experiements signed an informed consent form that explained the procedures, risks, and benefits, let them know they could quit at any time without prejudice (fewer than 10 percent did), and informed them that their results would be published. The Institutional Research Board, Committee on Human Subject Research, of the University of California at Santa Cruz approved the experimental design, oversaw the research, and helped assure compliance with relevant provisions of the Health Insurance Portability and Accountability Act (HIPAA).

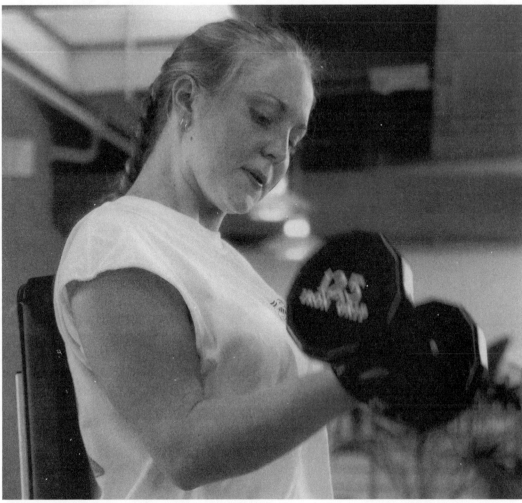

Photo by D. T. Wood

Sarah Pinneo nears the end of her IBC workout.

using all seven metrics on the exercise yardstick (chapter 2). In each experiment, male and female, the IBC and conventional exercise groups were matched initially for muscle strength, muscle endurance, and aerobic capacity (VO_{2max}), and they did their workouts at the same time of day to minimize extraneous variables.

Members of the IBC group did the advanced workout described in chapter 6, keeping their heart rate in the training window by cardio-accelerating between each set of weightlifting exercises. The conventional exercise group did the same types of exercise, and exactly the same resistance exercises, matched for total workload. The conventional exercise subjects rested between sets of weightlifting

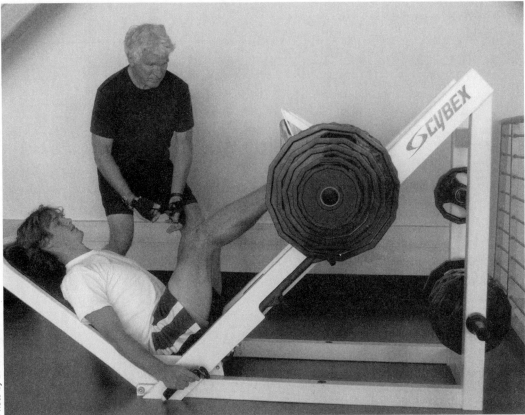

Eric Tozer, a member of the championship men's soccer team, tries
800 pounds on the leg press while I spot.

exercises, however, to keep their heart rate low. Both groups used the two other
elements of IBC described in chapter 1—integration of different exercise modes in
the same workout, and progression based on biofeedback—so in practice we limited our scientific evaluation to just one of the three elements of IBC, elevated
heart rate during resistance training.*

To test subjects, we made more than 100 separate measurements on every subject in both groups, IBC and conventional exercise, before and after their 10-week

---

* This limit was both conservative and necessary—conservative because it tests only one of the three elements of IBC, and necessary because otherwise we could not have separated out the effects of one variable (in this case elevated heart rate), which is the guiding purpose of a controlled scientific experiment.

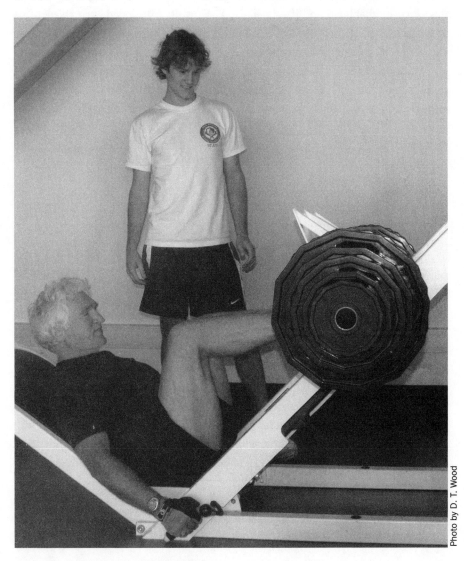

Eric spots me while I rep 800 pounds.

training program. In this process, we collected data representing every metric on the exercise yardstick as well as health and wellness indicators such as blood pressure. We also recorded dozens of measures of every workout for each athlete, including self-assessed DOMS and other pain, using the scales and workout logs described in chapter 6 and its appendix. The results astounded even those of us who already did IBC regularly. We'll highlight the women's results here because the sample size was larger; results from the men were generally compatible.

Lower body muscle strength* in these women athletes increased a remarkable 24 percent in the IBC group, and a respectable 17.7 percent in the conventional exercise group, over 10 weeks of training—a 35.6 percent advantage to IBC. Upper body strength increased a respectable 20 percent in both groups. These results show that IBC is up to one-third more effective in growing muscle strength, and suggest that the benefits over conventional exercise apply to muscles employed for cardio-driving, in this case the lower body.[†]

Muscle Endurance

Training effects on muscle endurance paralleled those for muscle strength, and the differences were more dramatic. We again analyzed results in two categories—lower and upper body—and measured endurance as the before-and-after differences in the maximum repetitions of each exercise at 50 percent (women) or 65 percent (men) of the one-repetition maximum weight. For the lower body, the endurance improvement of women in the IBC group was 31.6 percent, in comparison with 18.2 percent for the women who did conventional exercise—an IBC advantage of 73.6 percent. Once again, the differences in endurance for the upper body were not significant—both the IBC and conventional exercise subjects showed small increases that differed by an insignificant 2.9 percent. IBC therefore appears to increase both strength and endurance disproportionately and selectively in whatever muscles do the cardio-driving. This result dispels the interference effect (see the sidebar on page 50).

---

* We measured muscle strength by determining the standard one-repetition maximum (1-RM) for each of eight exercises, three for the lower body, and five for the upper body, before and after training. Lower body strength is the sum of 1-RM weights for three lower body exercises: leg press, leg extension, and leg flexion. Upper body strength is the sum of 1-RM weights for the lat pull-down, overhead press, arm curl, and triceps extensions.

† We hypothesize that the difference between lower and upper body results reflects the fact that cardio-driving was accomplished with lower body muscles (treadmill, stair-stepper, and step plyometrics). It would be interesting to repeat this experiment using upper body muscles for cardio-driving (rowing, arm ergometer). If the hypothesis is correct, the advantage would then appear for upper body strength. In the meantime, I have switched to a full-body cardio exercise, rowing, for my IBC workouts.

Aerobic Capacity, Cardiovascular Adaptation, and Blood Pressure

Aerobic capacity, or VO_{2max}, is the gold standard of physical fitness (chapter 2) and the best single index of longevity. Prior to the 10-week training program, the average VO_{2max} of the women athletes was slightly higher in the conventional exercise group (47.4) than the IBC group (43.8). Training increased the aerobic capacity of the IBC group by an average of 22.7 percent, however, while the group that did conventional exercise increased by 14 percent. IBC therefore produced a 63.2 percent greater gain in aerobic capacity, so by the end of the 10-week training period, the VO_{2max} of both groups was indistinguishable (53.9 for the IBC group, 54.1 for the conventional exercise group). IBC therefore produced at least two-thirds faster growth than the best conventional exercise prescription for this most important indicator of physical fitness.

Aerobic capacity is only one of several related indicators of cardiovascular health. Other indicators include cardiovascular adaptation—the steady decline in your average heart rate at any given exercise intensity as you get in better shape. In the male athletes, cardiovascular adaptation increased an astounding 150 percent faster in the IBC group than in the conventional exercise group. You will see the same cardiovascular adaptation in yourself during your IBC program, particularly if you keep workout logs. Look for this training effect as the steady decline in your average heart rate during the cardio phase of each IBC workout even though the level of the exercise stays the same or increases, or the constancy of heart rate despite increasing intensity of cardio exercise.

Blood pressure is another key indicator of cardiovascular health. High blood pressure, or hypertension is one of the strongest risk factors for heart disease. People who are hypertensive have a systolic pressure—the force of blood against the inner walls of vessels when the heart contracts—of 140 mm Hg or higher, and a diastolic pressure—the force when the heart is relaxed between beats—of 90 or higher. One in three Americans now have high blood pressure, and this proportion is increasing throughout the industrialized world at epidemic rates even in children. Pharmaceutical companies make fortunes every year marketing drugs to reduce blood pressure, and the heart disease that results from failure to control blood pressure is responsible for billions of dollars more in medical costs.

Many studies have already shown that exercise is effective in reducing blood pressure. A drop of 5–10 points in 10 weeks is typical for conventional exercise approaches. The women athletes in the IBC group showed a remarkable 17-point average drop in resting systolic blood pressure and a 10-point drop in resting diastolic pressure over the 10-week training program. In contrast, the conventional

Myth Buster 3: Is Cardio Really Dead?

THE MYTH: Cardio exercise interferes with strength training.

A generation of trainers, coaches, and bodybuilders has labored under the misapprehension that cardiovascular exercise—aerobics—is counterproductive to increases in muscle strength and mass. Just look at elite runners, they argued, who are in excellent cardio shape, but typically lean and wiry—even downright skinny—rather than layered with chiseled muscle.

It is a well-established tradition in bodybuilding to avoid cardio exercise before weightlifting, except for a brief warm-up. The reason: "You need to save your energy for the most important task at hand—lifting with intensity."[1] In view of the benefits of strength training for weight control, other observers have reflected that "weights might wipe out aerobics for good."[2]

The old recommendation to avoid combining cardio with resistance exercise was supported by the science of the time. A limited amount of older research appeared to suggest that combining cardiovascular exercise with strength training interfered with growth of muscle and strength—the so-called interference effect. More numerous and recent research studies, however, are documenting just the opposite, as are the studies described here.

The women we trained for 10 weeks with IBC gained an average of more than 4 pounds of lean, toned muscle. Individual women gained up to 10 pounds of sleek new muscle, and lost just as much fat, with no sign whatever of bulking up. The male athletes we trained showed similar gains—more than 3 pounds of new muscle on the average, and up to nearly 7 pounds individually.

Hold on—what about those lean elite runners? It turns out that they aren't skinny because of what they do—cardio exercise—but rather because of what they do not do—weightlifting. Put cardio together with weight training in the same workout, as in IBC, and both your heart and your muscles will get stronger far faster, and you'll shed more fat, too.

THE REALITY: Cardiovascular exercise enhances strength gains from weightlifting; conversely, separating these exercises loses that advantage.

The IBC Myth Buster

MYTH: Cardio exercise interferes with strength gains.

FACT: Integrating cardio exercise with weight training accelerates both strength and muscle gain.

exercise group showed an 11-point drop in resting systolic and diastolic pressure, in line with other studies on the relation between exercise and blood pressure. IBC therefore produced a 50 percent greater drop in resting systolic blood pressure in comparison with the best conventional exercise prescription.

We don't know why IBC selectively targeted systolic blood pressure, but whatever the explanation, an average drop in systolic blood pressure of 17 points in 10 weeks exceeds even extreme claims for blood pressure medications. Exercise at an elevated heart rate could therefore become a new tool for combating hypertension without drugs and the risks of their adverse effects. In the meantime, these results collectively show that IBC appears to strengthen aerobic capacity and related cardiovascular health indicators much faster than the best conventional exercise prescription.

Body Flexibility

Of all the universal dimensions of exercise, body flexibility is the most difficult to study. The problem is measurement reliability—few measures of flexibility are replicable across different trials or individuals. We used the two most widely accepted standards—the shoulder flexibility test and the YMCA sit-and-reach test. In the shoulder flexibility test, you raise one arm, lower the other, and then try to touch your hands behind your back. Then you reverse arms. The sum of the distance between your fingertips in the two trials is a rough index of shoulder flexibility. In the sit-and-reach test, you sit on the floor with your bare feet against a special box and lean forward as far as possible in one continuous, smooth movement. The forward reach distance is an approximate gauge of hamstring and trunk flexibility.

Prior to training, the women in the IBC group showed a mean separation of about ¾ inch between their fingertips in the shoulder flexibility test. After training, the mean value dropped to ¼ inch—a 70 percent improvement. In contrast, the group that did conventional exercise went from ½ inch of separation before training to 1 inch after—they actually became *less* flexible by 100 percent. IBC thus enjoyed a 170 percent advantage in shoulder flexibility. We don't know why flexibility declined in the conventional exercise group, but muscle soreness could play a role.

The results of the YMCA sit-and-reach test were similar, if less dramatic. Subjects in the IBC group showed an improvement of 8.4 percent, while subjects in the comparison group, who did conventional exercise, showed a smaller increase of 6.5 percent—a 28 percent advantage for IBC. Even though flexibility is the hardest metric on the exercise yardstick to assess quantitatively, these results nonetheless support the hypothesis that IBC increases body flexibility faster than the best conventional workout.

Body Composition

For many people, the whole point of exercise is to shed fat and gain muscle—in other words, to achieve a more healthy body composition. Women in the IBC group gained an average of 4.2 pounds of Fat Free Mass (FFM) over the 10 weeks of training, equivalent to nearly 0.5 pound of new muscle per athlete per week. The muscle gains of individual women in the IBC group ranged from a low of 0.1 pound to an astonishing high of 10 pounds. The latter corresponds to an increase of about 0.3 pound of solid new muscle *per workout*—the fastest rate of muscle gain we have ever seen in a drug-free training regime. Despite these remarkable gains in muscle mass, not one of the female subjects showed the slightest sign of bulking up. After training, their bodies instead appeared tighter, stronger, more toned, or more defined, depending on their individual physiology.

The comparison group that did conventional exercise, and rested between weightlifting exercises to keep their heart rate low, also gained muscle mass, but at less than half the rate of those who did IBC. The mean muscle gain in conventional exercise for women was 1.9 pounds, and ranged from negative 1.9 pounds (a loss of FFM) to a robust gain of 7 pounds. Recall that the only difference between the IBC and conventional group was heart rate during resistance training. These results show that applying just one of the three IBC elements, elevated heart rate during other exercise, produced twice the gain in muscle mass over the best conventional exercise prescription we could devise. The added effects of the other two IBC elements—integration of different exercise modes and progression based on biofeedback—remain untested, but they could amplify the IBC advantage even further.

The other side of the body composition coin is fat loss. We did not keep track of caloric intake in these experiments, and the athletes made no deliberate attempt to lose body weight, eating whatever they wanted during the 10-week training program. We were therefore amazed to discover that the IBC group lost an average of 2.7 pounds of fat per athlete, in comparison with a small net gain in body fat of 0.2 pound for the conventional exercise group. IBC burns more calories during workouts, but it also creates more muscle mass, which burns more calories between workouts, in comparison with the best conventional exercise prescription. IBC was therefore 300 percent more effective in shedding fat than the best conventional exercise prescription, and the fat loss occurred without deliberate calorie restriction.

Energy Systems Training

Determining changes in energy systems efficiency requires complex measurements on respiratory gases and blood chemistry, beyond the scope of our experiments.

Instead, we infer differences in energy systems using indirect indicators such as muscle strength and endurance (which use the first two energy gears), and aerobic capacity (which tests the third). By these measures, IBC exceeded the training effects of the best conventional exercise prescription by an estimated 50–100 percent.

The Fun Factor

The seventh metric on the exercise yardstick is the fun factor—how much you enjoy your exercise program. Although it's last on our list, it is first in importance—the more enjoyable your exercise program, the more likely you are to get it going and stay with it for a lifetime. To explore the fun factor, we did a separate study of 30 deconditioned college students (two-thirds female) who enrolled in a beginning physical education class at UCSC. Most of them had never exercised. This group represents a good cross section of young people new to exercise. We then trained these 30 students in seven different exercise programs, including indoor (gym-based) IBC.*

At the end of the quarter, after learning and doing the seven exercise programs, the students graded each program using the A–F scale. IBC won this competition handily, with an average grade of 3.8 on the 4-point scale, or an A-minus. Outdoor exercise was second, with a grade of B-plus. Put the two together—IBC plus outdoor exercise—and you can imagine how appealing the outdoor IBC workouts can be (chapter 7).

We also invited these 30 students to comment on their favorite workout, and to say why it was most enjoyable for them (testimonial evidence). Here is an unedited sampling of some of their replies.

- "Integrated Body Conditioning was my favorite because I pushed myself hard and I wasn't sore or tired the next day. I also felt like I got more out of my weight training with the high heart rate."
- "I liked [IBC]. I was very active and positive the whole day."
- "Integrated Body Conditioning. I really felt great when we were finished. Also it makes the time you spend lifting and running go by fast. It helped me breathe while I was lifting."
- "Integrated Body Conditioning because it was a great full-body workout and I felt like I got the best workout in this amount of time."
- "Integrated Body Conditioning because it kept me in constant motion and kept my heart rate up. I was continuously doing something."

* The other six protocols were: (1) basic circuit training, (2) triple weightlifting sets for endurance training (30/20/10 repetitions), (3) triple sets for strength, (4) stability ball exercises, (5) outdoor exercises using body weight, and (6) functional integrated strength (multijoint exercises).

- "Integrated Body Conditioning—felt like I actually got a good workout, wasn't ever standing around."
- "I like combining cardio and weight training. It feels more productive than the basic circuit."

Delayed Onset Muscle Soreness

Perhaps the most important advantage of IBC is that the superior results described above come with little or no Delayed Onset Muscle Soreness (DOMS). Not only does IBC enable you to grow faster, but your body also recovers faster. We documented reduced soreness by recording DOMS in every athlete for every exercise in every workout, using the Rating of Perceived Pain or Borg scale (chapter 6). We calibrated this subjective measure by recording DOMS following one-repetition maximum trials before conditioning started. The IBC group and the conventional exercise group reported about the same DOMS levels for each exercise, showing that they understood and implemented the subjective Borg scale similarly.

As the participants then did their three workouts every week, we entered the data from each workout into a computer for immediate graphical display. The graph of self-reported DOMS (figure 3.1) therefore emerged day by day.

In the male athletes (figure 3.1), it took a couple of workouts before DOMS dropped in the IBC group. By the third workout, the IBC participants reported one-fifth to one-tenth the muscle soreness of their counterparts who did the same resistance exercises at lower heart rates. The female athletes who did IBC showed a big difference in DOMS from the beginning. Further research is needed to learn whether there is a genuine gender difference in DOMS reduction using IBC. In the meantime, these findings confirm the hypothesis, based originally on case studies, that elevating heart rate during resistance training largely eliminates muscle soreness.

The UCSC Women's Soccer Team

In the 2003–2004 regular soccer season, before training with IBC, the women's soccer team had a 9:7:1 record (won/lost/tied) and was unranked. This year, after training with IBC, these women athletes were undefeated in pre-season play against opponents in their division. At this writing, halfway through their regular soccer season, the team enjoys a 9:2:1 record (won/lost/tied) in regular play and is currently ranked fourth in the West Region.

Here is a small selection of what these women athletes had to say about IBC:

- "I feel like I am in the best shape of my life. I can't believe the difference it has made on the field."

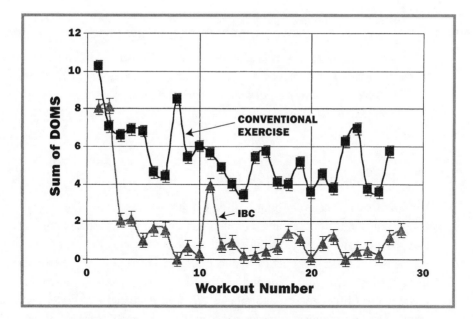

FIGURE 3.1 Sum of self-reported Delayed Onset Muscle Soreness (DOMS) in the group that did conventional exercise in comparison with those who did IBC. DOMS was summed over nine resistance exercises and averaged for each workout. The IBC group reported one-fifth to one-tenth the DOMS. Vertical bars = two standard errors of the population mean.

- "My favorite aspect of this program is the integration of cardio with weight training. The benefits are astounding—it's a method I will definitely incorporate into my future fitness regimes."
- "Other fitness programs I've done had room to improve or not. This program helped me push myself as far as I could go."
- "My first realization of my vast strength improvement occurred in a pickup soccer game when I pushed a man a foot taller than me off the ball with ease. I'm not sure which of us was more amazed. . . ."
- "My teammates have told me they have never seen me play better."
- "Every time I step on the field I feel a lot more confident, like the other team doesn't have a chance now."
- "It is one thing to get lost in this engaging workout and feel my gains, but it is another to see my appearance change so rapidly. I have learned to respect my body for the work it can accomplish."

The coach of the women's soccer team, Michael Runeare, said this at the end of the program and a perfect pre-season against Division III opponents:

The IBC program has been a huge success for the women's soccer team. Physically, it has increased their endurance and strength, particularly in their ability to recover from strenuous efforts. Mentally, participating in the program has increased their confidence and success on the field and enabled our team to play at another level. I highly recommend IBC for any athlete looking for a competitive edge.

The UCSC Men's Soccer Team

Winning may not be everything—attitude is just as important. The two are certainly compatible, however, and for most people winning is more fun. For competitive athletes, winning with attitude is the name of the game. Even if you are not a competitive athlete, the practical applications of exercise programs are important in evaluating them. You want and deserve the greatest possible return on your investment of time, energy, and money. We have evaluated IBC performance in terms of its impact on game performance of the UCSC men's soccer team in Division III of the National Collegiate Athletic Association (NCAA). The comparison illuminates the potent impact of IBC on athletic performance—and, by implication, on your own performance and results from your IBC program.

In the 2002 season, before they trained with IBC, the men's soccer team won 11 games, lost 5, and tied 2, a win percentage of 61 percent. Not bad, but the team was not ranked nationally; nor was it ranked in the NCAA West Region. Following three months of off-season training and a summer IBC maintenance program, the team's 2003 record was 21 wins and 2 losses, for a win percentage of 91 percent. The team ranked first in the West Region, and fifth in the nation in both the NCAA and Adidas National and Regional Rankings. These are the highest rankings ever for a UCSC soccer team. Coach Paul Holocher was named the NCAA and Adidas 2003 West Region Coach of the Year, while two team members—Matt King and Dan Chamberlain—were elected to the West Region All-American soccer team.

Perhaps the most telling aspect of the soccer team's performance is in goals scored and scored against. In the 2002 season, before IBC, the team scored 42 goals, while in the 2003 season, following off-season training in IBC, they scored 87 (table 3.1)—third in the nation. That's an increase of 107 percent! At the same time, goals scored against the team declined 25 percent, from eight in 2002 to six in 2003–2004. Dan Chamberlain, our West Region All-American goalie, had the fewest goals scored against him of anyone in West Region Division III play. The ratio of goals scored to goals scored against went from 5:1 in the 2002 soccer season, prior to training in IBC, to 15:1 after. The scoring effectiveness of the soccer team following IBC training therefore showed a 300 percent improvement.

A closer look at scoring by game half (table 3.1) illustrates the potential training effect of IBC on energy systems. Before training (2002), the team scored 4.25 goals in the second half for every goal scored by the opposition. After training in IBC (2003), they scored 11.25 goals in the second half for every goal scored by the opposition. Team scoring effectiveness in the second half therefore showed a 264 percent improvement. The reason for the heightened scoring prowess was plain to spectators—most opponents simply could not keep up with these superbly conditioned athletes during the second half of each game.

Team statistics for all intercollegiate athletic teams, including men's soccer, are available on the website of the NCAA.* The UCSC team was unranked nationally prior to IBC training, and ranked fifth in the nation after (table 3.2). The team was unranked in all categories in the 1999–2000 soccer season, but made a quantum leap in ranking after training in IBC.

IBC naturally does not deserve all the credit for the achievements of the UCSC men's soccer team. West Regional Soccer Coach of the Year Paul Holocher went to heroic lengths to grow his team, and it is impossible to measure the impact of such inspired coaching. The soccer team also enjoyed tremendous depth from excellent and in some cases elite athletes. So how can we realistically assess the contributions of IBC?

In every successful team, three qualities converge—conditioning, motivation, and skills. In theory, IBC is limited to conditioning. On the other hand, both the players and the coaches of the men's soccer team discovered that the conditioning of the team as an integrated system using IBC not only increased the strength and endurance of individual athletes, but also generated team camaraderie that carried onto the field. The superb physical conditioning of individual players also increased general team motivation, by revealing to members of the team their physical capacities, and provided a stronger basis for skill development. You can learn and execute soccer skills such as dribbling, passing, heading, cutting, and footwork far more effectively when you are in the best possible physical condition. The three components of team success—conditioning, motivation, skills—in fact come as a package, and the superb physical conditioning achieved with IBC had a powerful carryover impact on the other two components of team success.

* Go to www.NCAA.org and click on "News & Publications/Sports Statistics/Men's Soccer/Division III, Team Statistics and Archived" for the original data summarized in table 3.2.

TABLE 3.1
SCORING BY SEASON, TEAM, AND HALF, UCSC VERSUS ALL OPPONENTS

Season	Team	First Half	Second Half	Total
2002 ↓ IBC training ↓ 2003	UCSC Goals	25	17	42
	Opponent Goals	4	4	8
	UCSC Goals	42	45	87
	Opponent Goals	2	4	6

Goals scored by the UCSC men's soccer team increased by more than 100 percent after training with Integrated Body Conditioning (prior to the 2003 season), while second-half scoring effectiveness increased by 264 percent.

TABLE 3.2
NATIONAL RANKINGS OF THE UCSC MEN'S SOCCER TEAM, 2001–2004

Team Statistic	2001–2002 (before IBC)	2002–2003 (before IBC)	2003–2004 (after IBC)
Scoring Offense	<30	<30	3
Goals Against	12	<30	9
Shutout Percentage	13	8	13
Won-Lost-Tied Percentage	30	7	3
Average Across Statistics	22	19	7

Following training in IBC, the mean ranking of the men's soccer team went from 19 to 7 in those categories of team statistics recorded by the NCAA and posted on its website. Averages across statistics were calculated conservatively by assigning a score of 31 to unranked statistics.

Perhaps the best indicator of the impact of IBC, however, comes from the comments of the coaches and players themselves. Team captain and NCAA West Region All-American goalie Dan Chamberlain, now a professional soccer player, said, "We couldn't have reached the national championships without Integrated Body Conditioning!" Matt King, also an NCAA West Region All-American, agreed: "IBC was a huge part of our national championship run." Here is a partial chronicle of what the other soccer players said about the role of IBC in their remarkable individual and team success, in their own, unedited words. Additional testimonials appear on the IBC website:

- "I got fit and increased my strength at the same time. I never felt sore, so it was easy to lift. The increased strength improved my game because I no longer got knocked off the ball."
- "The best aspect of the IBC training program was the soreness factor. Once we got into it I really never felt sore."
- "I really enjoyed the cardio aspect of the workout. I've never been in shape while doing a gym workout program."
- "The best thing about the IBC training program for me was being on a consistent program that was organized so that you could monitor your progress and meet higher goals."
- "I enjoyed the cardiovascular work between each lifting, but most of all I enjoyed my strength gain."
- "The logs keep you in check and you are able to track your progression. Strength increases greatly. I had a personal trainer before, but this program blew that away."
- "I saw in the post-testing, and just felt in my body, an extremely strong improvement in upper body strength. It was particularly effective for me to have the structure of coming in a few times a week for a long time, and because of that I was able to really improve."

At the end of the IBC program, the athletes evaluated their training program in comparison with other exercise programs or systems they had used. Most of these athletes had been in training since early youth, including soccer camps, personal trainers, and specialized physical training such as plyometrics, and yet three-quarters of them rated the IBC training system as the "Best I've Experienced." Here is what Coach Paul Holocher had to say at the end of the 2003 season:

There is no question IBC propelled us into the national championships. Our performance was light-years ahead of what we were able to accomplish last year. You don't often get a season like this, and IBC deserves a lot of the credit. I would not want to coach a team ever again without IBC as the foundation for our physical conditioning.

To their enormous credit, Coach Holocher and the men's soccer team had an even better 2004 season, finishing second in the nation in their division.

The Path Ahead

Science usually raises more questions than it answers, and our research on IBC is no exception. The results to date support the conclusion that IBC is the most comprehensive, effective, and efficient conditioning program you can use. In these controlled scientific experiments, IBC was consistently superior to the best conventional exercise prescription by every measure and produced little or no muscle soreness. But why does IBC work so well? Why does your heart strengthen so fast and your blood pressure drop so dramatically? Why does IBC increase strength in the muscles used to cardio-drive? How is it even possible to add muscle mass so fast? Why does the IBC make you feel so energetic, and why don't you get sore?

We don't have the answers to these and many other questions about IBC. Moreover, our conclusions come from studies on slightly more than 200 subjects, mainly college students. Medical science typically accepts results only after replication by different laboratories on diverse populations of hundreds and even thousands of subjects. Answering the unanswered questions and extending these studies to broader and larger populations will be tasks for future research, which this book will hopefully initiate.

In the meantime, based on the results to date, IBC is now the foundation for training in all sports at the University of California at Santa Cruz, including the number-one-ranked men's tennis team. Although it will take years, and perhaps a generation, before the science is complete, the question in the meantime for *your* path is: Can you, or your team, afford to wait?

■ ■ ■

Your Miracle Workout Performance Manual

This is your three-step guide to IBC. Regardless of your fitness level, age, or preferences, you will find all you need here to follow the fastest, safest, most effective, and most enjoyable path to health and wellness (chapter 4), physical fitness (chapter 5), and peak performance (chapter 6). Go!

4

Your Beginning Miracle Workout

The beginning IBC program is ideal for you if you are new to exercise or have not exercised continuously for the past six months. It is the entry-level version of IBC that most people in good health can do. Even if you are an experienced exerciser, start here to learn the ABCs of IBC. You can graduate at your own pace to higher levels appropriate to your goals and abilities. The beginning IBC program may be appropriate for you even if you belong to a medically defined special population, although you may need to follow special precautions and exercise with the approval of your doctor (chapter 9).

The general goals of exercise fall into three broad categories: health and wellness, physical fitness, and peak athletic performance. The beginning IBC workout targets the first set, including weight control, feeling good, maintaining mobility, and managing everyday pain. You can achieve these goals in a 30-minute IBC workout three times a week with effort equivalent to a brisk walk. In the process, you will meet the U.S. surgeon general's minimum threshold for harvesting the health and wellness benefits of exercise. Then, if your goals remain focused on health and wellness, you can continue with variations on the beginning IBC program for as long as you wish, including your whole life—or you can step up to the next level.

Safety First

Be as sure as possible first that it is safe for you to do any exercise. Complete the PAR-Q form and Symptoms Questionnaire in the appendix to this chapter or on our website (www.MiracleWorkout.com; click on "Safety" and then "Beginning"). If you answer yes to any of the questions there, talk to your doctor before you begin to exercise or change your physical activity. If you are taking any cardio-active medication or nonfood substance, or anything that might interact adversely with exercise, talk with your doctor. If you have known cardiovascular, pulmonary, or metabolic disease, get your doctor's approval before you change your physical activity level. If during exercise you ever experience excessive shortness of breath, pain in your chest or arm, heart arrhythmia, head pain or dizziness, stop exercising immediately and get professional advice.

If you answered no to all the questions on the two forms, you are ready to go. According to the guidelines of the American College of Sports Medicine (ACSM), if you are in good health, it is safe at any age to do moderate exercise, as in the beginning IBC program, without a special medical exam and without a doctor-supervised exercise test. If your exercise intensity ever exceeds moderate as defined below, however, use the more stringent safety procedures described in chapters 5 and 6. Above all, take comfort in the consensus among physicians and exercise professionals that it is far safer to exercise than not.

Hydrate Early and Often

Water is essential to life, and drinking plenty during exercise is necessary to reap all the benefits of exercise. The Gatorade Company conducted a study a few years ago showing that fewer than half of all exercisers drink enough fluid during their workouts. When you exercise, you speed up all the biochemical reactions that underlie life, and you sweat, which means you lose water faster. You need to replace this water in order to both support the accelerated biochemical reactions induced by your workout and sustain the increased sweat response that keeps your body temperature within safe limits.

There is another, less obvious consequence of dehydration. Sweat comes mainly from the fluid part of your blood, the plasma. Unless you replenish this liquid, plasma volume declines and your blood literally gets thicker. Your heart then has to work harder to feed and cleanse your muscles, and the process is less efficient. Proper hydration avoids the thick blood syndrome and cleanses your body—a kind of bath from the inside out, the full-body flush (chapter 5). You receive this benefit in direct proportion to how much you sweat, which is more at the advanced IBC levels, but you will harvest some benefits at the beginning level.

To avoid dehydration, drink early and often. Consume 8–12 ounces of water 20 minutes before you start to exercise and then take frequent drinks during your workout. A good rule of thumb for hydration during exercise is to drink a quart of water per hour per 100 pounds of body weight, in addition to your pre-workout drink. If you wait until you are thirsty, it is already too late—thirst signals come from having too little water in your body's system. It is hard to drink too much water—the average person has to drink more than 10 quarts before water intoxication (hyponatremia) occurs. High-performance athletes who drink large quantities of water without replacing electrolytes may be at risk from water intoxication, as are people who are on diuretic medication for hypertension.

There is an easy test of whether you drink enough. Weigh yourself before your workout, and then again immediately after. Assuming you were hydrated correctly at the start of your workout, you should weigh at least the same when you finish, signifying that you have replaced all of the water released during exercise. Carry a calibrated water bottle with you when you exercise, and record the amount of water you consume during each workout. Then adjust your water intake as needed, determined by the before-and-after weight test. Once you determine your optimum water intake for a given exercise intensity and duration, it stays about the same unless your weight changes dramatically.

Drinking plenty of water does not interfere with either fat loss or weight control. The high fluid flux does increase your exposure to whatever impurities may be in the water, making it even more important to ensure water quality. Normal tap water contains chlorine, which may be beneficial for public health, but is nonetheless toxic to individuals. You can avoid it by drinking bottled springwater or filtered water.

The Blueprint for Your Beginning IBC Program

You can do IBC anywhere—at home, outdoors (chapter 7), in a gym, or in a health club. In this and the next two chapters, however, we'll focus on the gym workout to ensure consistency of description across levels. Then we'll develop the other options (chapter 7). If you think a gym membership is too expensive, think again—it can save you money in the long run (see the sidebar on the following page).

Approach the fully integrated IBC workout at your own pace in three steps (figure 4.1)—cardio, cardiorom, and the final, fully integrated cardiolift. Step 1, cardio, prepares your heart and your phosphorous and aerobic energy systems. Step 2, cardiorom, limbers your joints, strengthens your tendons and ligaments,

Myth Buster 4: Too Much Money

THE MYTH: Exercising costs too much money. I can't afford it.

Think that gym membership, or heart monitor, or that set of barbells, costs too much? Unlike most exercise programs, you can do IBC for next to nothing. Even if you splurge on fancy workout clothes, equipment, and a gym membership, you should still be forking out, on average, less than $100 per month. That's not bad in comparison with the alternatives.

A single day in the hospital can cost several thousand dollars. Cardiac rehabilitation exercise training following a heart attack costs $9,200 per year. If you are one of the 45 million Americans who don't have health insurance, that money comes straight out of your pocket. If IBC spares you or someone who you love just one day per year in the hospital, that's a saving of several tens of thousands of dollars over a lifetime.

In a broader societal context, workers' compensation costs are soaring, straining many businesses, small and large. A four-year study on employees of the Xerox Corporation showed that 85 percent of all workers' compensation costs are associated with excess health risk—which decline dramatically with exercise. The savings per person was $1,238. If you are a business owner or manager, what could an exercise program do for your bottom line?

Health care costs in the United States exceed a trillion dollars per year and consume an estimated 14 percent of gross domestic product. That number is likely to go up dramatically as baby boomers come of age. Most of those medical and health care costs result from diseases whose risks decline dramatically with exercise. Obesity alone accounts for more than 10 percent of the total bill, and is rising. If your IBC program eliminates just half those costs, the average family of four would save a whopping $10,000 every year. The savings could pay for your college education, or those of your children or grandchildren, or we could pay down the national debt in a few years!

THE REALITY: You cannot afford not to exercise. Exercise does not cost money, it saves it, for individuals and society at large.

The IBC Myth Buster

MYTH: Exercise, including IBC, is too expensive.

FACT: IBC saves money, and lots of it, over the short and long terms.

FIGURE 4.1
THE THREE-STEP BEGINNING IBC PROGRAM MADE SIMPLE

1. **Prerequisites.** Good health, no cardiovascular or other contraindicated symptoms (see appendix, or go to www.MiracleWorkout.com and click on "Safety" and then "Beginning").
2. **Intensity.** Moderate exercise only.
3. **Description.** Three steps: two preparatory and one integrated.

Step 1: Cardio (preparatory)

1. **Goal.** 30 minutes of moderate cardio exercise in complete comfort.
2. **Method.** Self-paced, progressive aerobic (cardio) exercise.
3. **Time.** 30 minutes per workout, three workouts per week, for two to four weeks.

Step 2: Cardiorom (preparatory, partially integrated)

1. **Goal.** Integration of ROM with moderate cardio exercise.
2. **Method.** Alternate moderate cardio and ROM exercise.
3. **Time.** 30 minutes per workout, three workouts per week, for two to four weeks.

Step 3: Cardiolift (fully integrated)

1. **Goal.** Integration of weightlifting with moderate cardio exercise, followed by ROM cooldown.
2. **Method.** Alternate cardio and weightlifting exercises with a terminal ROM cooldown.
3. **Time.** 30 minutes per workout, three workouts per week, until maintenance stage or graduation to the intermediate level.

and readies your body system for resistance training. Step 3, cardiolift, is an easy, short, and fully integrated workout that adds resistance training to your repertoir, developing muscles, bones, and your anaerobic energy system. This three-step approach will carry you through your IBC program in comfort and safety, and keep you engaged and growing until you achieve your desired body weight and exercise goals.

You can remain in the third, fully integrated cardiolift stage for as long as you like and reap many of the health and wellness benefits of IBC. Alternatively, use your newfound conditioning as a launching pad to the intermediate IBC program. To get there, you will learn to listen to your body—the practical application of body consciousness—and use this biofeedback to guide the intensity of your IBC workout and your rate of progression. Reliance on biofeedback is one of the three elements of IBC (chapter 1) that helps you develop so quickly and safely.

Three Elements of Biofeedback

Biofeedback is body signals made conscious. You will use three forms of biofeedback during IBC workouts: heart rate, perceived exertion, and perceived pain—or, more accurately, the absence of pain, which is the goal. You monitor your heart rate to keep your exercise intensity at the moderate level, defined as 55–69 percent of your maximum heart rate (table 4.1). Estimate your maximum heart rate by subtracting your age from 220. If you are 50, for example, your estimated maximum heart rate is 220 – 50, or 170. Take 55 percent of that to find the lower boundary of your heart rate training window (in our example, 93.5), and 69 percent to get

---

TABLE 4.1
HEART RATE TRAINING WINDOWS FOR DIFFERENT EXERCISE INTENSITIES BASED ON THE MAXIMUM HEART RATE METHOD
(Maximum heart rate = 220 – age in years)

Exercise Intensity Level	Percent of Maximum Heart Rate (Range)
Very light	<35%
Light	35–54%
Moderate	55–69%
Hard (vigorous)	70–89%
Very hard (heavy)	≥90%
Maximal	100%

From American College of Sports Medicine, *ACSM's Guidelines for Exercise Testing and Prescription,* sixth edition (Philadelphia: Lippincott Williams & Wilkins, 2000), table 7-2, p. 150. Adapted originally from M. L. Pollock, G. A. Gaesser, J. D. Butcher, et al. "The Recommended Quantity and Quality of Exercise for Developing and Maintaining Cardiorespiratory and Muscular Fitness, and Flexibility in Healthy Adults." *Med Sci Sports Exerc* 30 (1998), pp. 975–991. Copyright © 2000 by American College of Sports Medicine. Reproduced by permission of Lippincott Williams & Wilkins.

TABLE 4.2
MODERATE EXERCISE HEART RATE TRAINING WINDOWS FOR DIFFERENT AGES BASED ON THE MAXIMUM HEART RATE METHOD

Age (years)	Maximum Heart Rate (220 – age)	Moderate Heart Rate Training Window(BPM)
10	210	115–145
20	200	110–140
30	190	105–130
40	180	100–125
50	170	95–115
60	160	90–110
70	150	85–105
80	140	75–95
90	130	70–90
100	120	65–85

BPM = Beats per Minute. All ranges are rounded to the nearest 5, to make them easier to remember. The ranges shown assume you are not taking medications or substances that may influence heart rate up or down, or otherwise interact adversely with moderate exercise. If in doubt, consult your doctor.

the upper boundary (117.3). Round all values to the nearest five Beats per Minute (BPM) to make them easier to remember. For the 50-year-old, the moderate-intensity heart rate window is thus 95–115 BPM. After you calculate your heart rate training window, confirm that it is in the correct range from the decadal values in table 4.2.

Once you have determined your cardiovascular training window, the next step is to stay within it while you exercise, using one of three options: a heart monitor, the talk test, or pulse measurement. By far the most accurate is the heart monitor. It consists of two parts, a transmitter attached to an elastic strap that fits comfortably around your chest just beneath the breasts, and a receiver strapped to your wrist that displays your heart rate continuously. The simplest models show only instantaneous heart rate and cost around $50. More advanced models also record your exercise time, the time spent in your heart rate training window, your average heart rate, and the number of Kilocalories burned, and cost upward of $100. If there is a chance that you will eventually move to the intermediate or advanced levels of IBC, your best choice is the more advanced heart monitor.*

The second way to tell when you are exercising moderately is the talk test. If you are breathing hard but can carry on a multisentence conversation, you are probably exercising moderately. A moderate-intensity workout is therefore termed conversational exercise. If you are huffing and puffing so hard that you can only utter brief sentences and must then get back to breathing, you are probably exercising vigorously. The talk test is surprisingly accurate, and what it lacks in precision it makes up for in simplicity. On the other hand, you must talk to implement it, which can raise eyebrows if you're exercising alone. Once you advance to the vigorous intensity of the intermediate level, you may not wish to talk much during your workout.

The third way to tell if you are exercising moderately is to measure your pulse by hand. Place the two forefingers of your left hand on the radial artery in your right wrist, or on the carotid artery in your neck, and count the number of heartbeats in a 10-second period. Start the count at zero rather than one for accuracy, and multiply by six to get your approximate heart rate in BPM. The downside of the pulse method is that you have to interrupt your exercise frequently to measure your heart rate. If you can afford a heart monitor, you will find the precision and convenience worth the expense.

The second and third biofeedback signals that you will use are perceived exertion and perceived pain. Monitor these signals continuously when you exercise, and use them to regulate the intensity of your workout and to determine when to progress, which keeps you advancing at your own comfortable, safe pace. Both perceived exertion and perceived pain are determined conveniently using the same scale, developed by Dr. Gunnar Borg and also called the Borg scale (figure 4.2).

The Rating of Perceived Exertion (RPE) scale has found use primarily in a clinical setting, but there is a sound scientific reason for using it to regulate your workout. RPE is directly proportional to the buildup of muscle fatigue products in your blood during exercise. Although RPE is a subjective measure of exercise effort, it has an objective foundation. Our research shows that different groups of exercisers rate perceived exertion and perceived pain from a common exercise experience almost identically.

---

* You can purchase a heart monitor at your local sporting goods store or online at www.power-systems.com or www.amazon.com. The entry-level heart monitor is equivalent to the Polar A3, while a more advanced model that satisfies most needs is equivalent to the Polar A5.

FIGURE 4.2
THE RATING OF PERCEIVED EXERTION (RPE) AND RATING OF PERCEIVED PAIN (RPP) SELF-MEASURING SCALE

Use this qualitative scale to assess how much exertion your exercise or workout requires and to minimize pain. Add to your workload in your next workout (progress) only if your Rating of Perceived Exertion (RPE) is *strong* or less, and your Rating of Perceived Pain (RPP) is *weak* or less.

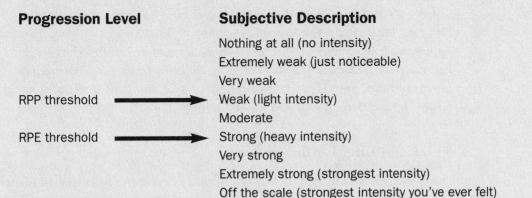

Progression Level	Subjective Description
	Nothing at all (no intensity)
	Extremely weak (just noticeable)
	Very weak
RPP threshold ⟶	Weak (light intensity)
	Moderate
RPE threshold ⟶	Strong (heavy intensity)
	Very strong
	Extremely strong (strongest intensity)
	Off the scale (strongest intensity you've ever felt)

Instructions for Use

RPE: "During the exercise . . . pay close attention to how hard you feel the exercise work rate is. This feeling should reflect your total amount of exertion and fatigue, combining all sensations and feelings of physical stress, effort, and fatigue. Don't concern yourself with any one factor such as leg pain, shortness of breath, or exercise intensity, but try to concentrate on your total, inner feeling of exertion. Evaluate your exertion using the scale above. Try not to underestimate or overestimate your feelings of exertion; be as accurate as you can."

RPP: "During the exercise . . . pay close attention to any pain you may feel anywhere in your body, including muscle soreness, joint, or trunk pain. Concentrate on the pain and estimate its intensity using the above scale. Try not to underestimate or overestimate your feeling of pain; be as accurate as you can."

Based on Gunnar Borg. *G. Borg's Perceived Exertion and Pain Scales* (Champaign, IL: Human Kinetics, 1998). Adapted with author permission.

The IBC Method of Progression

Recall the third element of IBC (chapter 1): Progress according to how your body feels. Add to your workout time or effort or move up to the next level when your Rating of Perceived Exertion (RPE) is *strong* or less, and your Rating of Perceived Pain (RPP) is *weak* or less. Otherwise, repeat the same workout at the same intensity and workload. You will use of this method of progression repeatedly at both a macro-scale, to advance from one preparatory step to the next as you ramp up to the cardiolift stage, and at the micro-scale, to regulate progress in individual weightlifting exercises.

This method of progression determines your rate of progress at every level of IBC, ensuring that you grow as quickly, comfortably, and safely as possible. There are just two critical values to remember—*strong* is your RPE threshold for advancing, and *weak* is your RPP threshold (figure 4.2). If either your perceived exertion or your perceived pain exceeds these thresholds, repeat your most recent workout, weight, or repetitions in your next exercise session.

The Beginning Cardio Workout

Spend a preparatory session in your health club learning and practicing all the options available for aerobic or cardiovascular exercise. Motorized options include the treadmill, the stair-stepper, the elliptical trainer, the stationary cycle, and the rowing machine. Most exercisers find the treadmill best for cardio-driving, but it also has the greatest impact on joints, which can be problematic for heavier or older exercisers. The stair-stepper and elliptical stepper are good cardio-accelerators, and easier on the joints. Some steppers have moving handgrips that engage the upper body, giving a better overall workout. Stationary cycling is perhaps the least effective cardio-driver, because you don't support your full body weight, but cycling is also comfortable and familiar and works well at the beginning level. The rowing machine provides the best full-body cardio workout but requires strong hands, wrists, and forearms.

Nonmotorized options for cardio-driving are useful for those occasions when the motorized machines are crowded, and for group, home, or outdoor workouts. They include the step-up platform or box, Bosu Ball, jogging or running in place, jumping in place, jumping rope, calisthenics such as jumping jacks, and more. Your gym may already have the equipment, or you can buy it from a sporting goods store or catalog (try www.power-systems.com) for less than $100 and, if your gym management approves, bring it with you to the gym for cardio-acceleration. The employees of your health club or gym can help you learn all of these aerobic exercise options.

Now you're ready. You are dressed for exercise, took a big drink 20 minutes ago, and have your water bottle and sweat towel in hand. Select your favorite cardio-driver and start your aerobics. Monitor your heart rate as it climbs during the first few minutes of exercise into your moderate cardiovascular training window (tables 4.1 and 4.2). Your cardio workout then becomes a little like a video game where you keep the race car on the track by adjusting the steering wheel, but instead it's your heart rate that you are holding within your training window by adjusting the intensity of your aerobic exercise. You are unlikely to experience any pain. If you do, and if it feels greater than weak, stop exercising and figure out its cause with professional or medical advice as required. Avoid the unnecessary risk of continuing to exercise if you feel any significant pain that you do not understand thoroughly.

Consider this first session of your IBC program as a practice run. Your initial purpose is to learn how to use your heart monitor to stay in your heart rate window for 5 or 10 minutes. When you finish this practice workout, do some light stretching and bending to cool down, using ROM exercises shown in figure 4.4. During the cooldown, keep your heart rate near your active rest level, defined for the beginning level as the lower limit of your moderate exercise heart rate window (55 percent of your maximum heart rate; see table 4.1). If you are 60 years of age, for example, your active rest heart rate for your cooldown will be about 90 BPM. The cooldown is important because it keeps your circulation flowing properly until you have recovered your normal resting breathing and heart rates. The cooldown should last at least five minutes.

Approach the goal of 30 continuous minutes of aerobic exercise in incremental steps and at your own pace. You achieve this by adding time in five-minute blocks to your moderate cardio exercise routine when you feel comfortable—that is, when your RPE for the workout is *strong* or less and your RPP is *weak* or less. Figure 4.3 outlines a representative hypothetical cardio workout to illustrate the IBC method of progression.

In the first couple of sessions of the cardio phase, you will master the heart monitor, the art of staying in your moderate heart rate training window, keeping your heart rate at the active rest level during your cooldown, and applying the IBC method of progression. Continue this process—exercise, self-evaluate, advance or repeat—until you can remain comfortably in your training window for 30 minutes with perceived exertion no greater than *strong* and perceived pain no greater than *weak.*

How long it takes to achieve the 30-minute milestone depends mainly on your initial physical condition and on how often you exercise. You can safely do moderate cardiovascular exercise every day, so if you exercise five times per week and if you progress 5 minutes each session, you'll reach the 30-minute milestone in less

FIGURE 4.3
SAMPLE BEGINNING CARDIO WORKOUT PROGRAM ILLUSTRATING THE IBC METHOD OF PROGRESSION

Here's a hypothetical cardio workout at the beginning level that illustrates how to progress using the IBC method.

Monday, Workout 1: Do your favorite cardio (aerobic) exercise until your heart rate enters the moderate training window (55–69 percent of your maximum heart rate), and keep it there for five minutes. Let's say your biofeedback was: RPE, *very strong;* RPP, *weak.*

Wednesday, Workout 2: Because your RPE in workout 1 exceeded *strong,* repeat workout 1—do another five-minute cardio workout. Biofeedback in this workout: RPE, *moderate;* RPP, *weak.*

Friday, Workout 3: Because your RPE in workout 2 was *strong* or less, and your RPP was *weak* or less, add 5 minutes to your cardio workout for a new time of 10 minutes. Biofeedback: RPE, *strong;* RPP, *weak.*

Monday, Workout 4: Since your RPE in workout 3 was *strong* or less, and RPP was *weak* or less, add 5 minutes to your moderate cardio workout for a new exercise time of 15 minutes. In this workout, however, let's suppose you experience a moderate side stitch at the end. Biofeedback: RPE, *strong;* RPP, *moderate.*

Wednesday, Workout 5: RPE the last time was *strong* or less, but RPP was *moderate,* which exceeds *weak* or less, so repeat the last workout by doing 15 minutes of moderate aerobic exercise. Biofeedback: RPE, *moderate;* RPP, *weak.*

Friday, Workout 6: The progression method adds 5 minutes, for a total moderate cardio workout of 20 minutes. Biofeedback: RPE, *strong;* RPP, *weak.*

Monday, Workout 7: Add 5 minutes, for a total workout of 25 minutes. Biofeedback: RPE, *strong;* RPP, *none.*

Wednesday, Workout 8: Add 5 minutes, for a total workout time of 30 minutes of moderate aerobic exercise. Biofeedback: RPE, *strong;* RPP, *none.* Congratulations, you are ready for the next stage!

This hypothetical exerciser has completed the cardio phase in eight workouts rather than the minimum of six, because of the two repeated workouts.

than a week. If you exercise three times per week and progress every session, you will reach the 30-minute goal in less than two weeks. It should take at most a few weeks before you're ready to graduate to the cardiorom phase.

When you reach the 30-minute milestone, you may be surprised to find that it feels nearly as easy as the 5 or 10 minutes of your first workout. The fact that you are comfortable exercising moderately and continuously for 30 minutes is an important milestone. Moderate exercise for 30 minutes provides many of the health benefits of exercise, including reduced risk of cardiovascular disease and longer, higher-quality life. For many people, such as deconditioned older seniors who have never before exercised, this may represent a satisfactory end point. On the other hand, you are now poised to advance to the cardiorom phase and harvest the additional health and wellness benefits that come from full-body flexibility.

The Beginning Cardiorom Workout

The second step of the three-step beginning IBC program, cardiorom, integrates bending and stretching into your 30-minute moderate cardio workout. Your goal is to strengthen your heart further while you attain the body flexibility needed to perform moderate resistance exercises in the third step. Cardiorom achieves these goals by alternating cardio with ROM exercises. Simply elevate your heart rate into your moderate training window with your favorite aerobic exercises, and then stretch and bend while your heart rate is elevated. Use the basic Range of Motion (ROM) exercises in figure 4.4, which include bending and stretching around each primary joint (the shoulders and hips) and each secondary joint (the knees and elbows).

You are now ready to integrate ROM exercises with cardiovascular exercise. Copy figure 4.4 or print it from www.MiracleWorkout.com in 8½-by-11-inch format (click on "Exercises"), and attach it to a clipboard to prop up in your ROM exercise area. Your gym should have an area set aside for stretching and bending exercises, stocked with individual rubber or foam floor mats for comfort and support, and roomy enough to let you stretch out on the floor without getting whacked by a dumbbell or bumping other exercisers. Take that large drink of water about 20 minutes before you begin.

Start your cardiorom with a five-minute aerobic warm-up at moderate intensity, and move directly to your first ROM exercise while your heart rate is still elevated into your moderate heart rate training window. Using a wall mirror or partner for feedback, stretch into the position shown in ROM exercise 1 of figure 4.4—the knee flexor (hamstring) stretch—and hold the position for 15 seconds. If you have trouble lifting your leg to a vertical position, use your hands to help out,

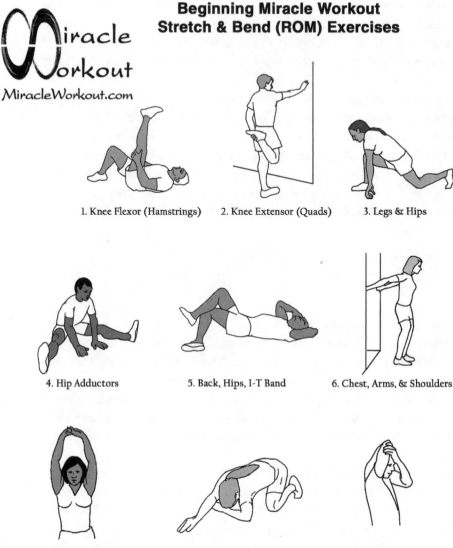

Beginning Miracle Workout
Stretch & Bend (ROM) Exercises

Miracle Workout
MiracleWorkout.com

1. Knee Flexor (Hamstrings)   2. Knee Extensor (Quads)   3. Legs & Hips

4. Hip Adductors   5. Back, Hips, I-T Band   6. Chest, Arms, & Shoulders

7. Shoulders, Arms   8. Upper Back (Lats)   9. Triceps

FIGURE 4.4 **Beginning IBC Stretch and Bend (ROM) Exercises** Here is a basic sequence of Range of Motion exercises that will enhance the flexibility of all your major joints—primary (the hips and shoulders) and secondary (the knees and elbows), as well as your core (abdomen and back). Hold the static positions shown for 15 seconds on each side of the body. Always warm up before stretching and bending to minimize the risk of injury.

and bend the opposite leg with foot flat on the floor as shown in figure 4.4. Note that for the first ROM exercise, you stretch each leg separately.

Your heart rate will decline during each ROM exercise, because stretching takes less effort than cardio exercise. Elevate it back into your moderate heart rate window with a short bout (about one minute) of cardiovascular exercise. Then perform your second ROM exercise (figure 4.4, exercise 2), while your heart rate is still elevated into your moderate heart rate window. You are now stretching the opposite muscle (quadriceps) from the one you stretched in exercise 1 (hamstrings), in accord with the balance principle.

You will immediately feel the IBC difference. The mild discomfort that normally attends stretching and bending is much less when your heart rate is elevated, and you may feel more limber than you imagined possible. As your workout proceeds, you will feel your three energy systems begin to ignite. You may even experience early hints of the runner's high. It's weaker during moderate than vigorous exercise, but look for signs starting about halfway through your cardiorom workout.

Several ROM exercises entail stretching each side of the body separately (figure 4.4, exercise 1). These exercises are unilateral—you stretch one side of your body at a time. In unilateral exercises, you will encounter a recurring issue in your IBC program—your heart rate may fall out of your training window before you get to the other side. To ensure that both sides benefit equally from cardio-driving, use one of two methods. First, elevate your heart rate to near the higher boundary of your moderate heart rate window. That will buy you a few more moments in your heart rate training window to complete both sides of your ROM exercise. Second, do a quick cardio-acceleration between stretching the two sides. This issue does not arise with bilateral ROM exercises (such as exercise 4 in figure 4.4, the hip stretch). Continue the process of alternating ROM with cardio until you have completed all nine of the ROM exercises shown in figure 4.4, or whatever other ROM exercise sequence you have chosen.

With a little experience, you'll be able to finish your beginning cardiorom workout in less than 30 minutes.* To advance through the cardiorom phase, work steadily higher in your moderate heart training rate window. For example, if you are 30 years of age, your moderate heart rate training window is 105–130 BPM

---

* Approximate timetable: 5 minutes for your warm-up, nine 1-minute intermittent cardio-acceleration bouts, nine ROM exercises averaging 30 seconds each, and 5 minutes for your cooldown, for a total of 23.5 minutes, plus some transaction time (such as walking between the cardio machine and your ROM station). If you do cardio bouts between stretching the two sides in a single ROM exercise, it'll take a little longer.

(table 4.2). As you move from one cardiorom workout to the next, move up gradually from 105 BPM to the midwindow value of 120 BPM. As always, advance when your perceived exertion is *strong* or less, and your perceived pain is *weak* or less. By the time you finish the cardiorom phase, you may be exercising near the lower boundary of vigorous exercise (table 4.1). You can also progress in the cardiorom stage by increasing the duration of your stretches, from the initial time of 15 seconds to 30 seconds.

The Beginning Cardiolift Workout

This third step of your three-step beginning IBC program integrates resistance training (weightlifting) into your cardio and ROM routine. The goals of the cardiolift phase of the beginning IBC workout are to learn basic resistance exercises, increase your overall body strength, and strengthen your heart to greater heights than cardio exercise alone can achieve. To reach these goals, do resistance exercises while your heart rate is elevated into your moderate heart rate training window. As in the cardiorom phase, keep your heart rate in your moderate training window by alternating short cardio-acceleration bouts with resistance exercises. Cool down at the end of the resistance exercises using your ROM routine alone, as a stand-alone series with no intermittent cardio-acceleration.

First learn your resistance exercises. Your investment in a health club or gym membership gives you access to a wide variety of equipment, as well as professional orientation and instruction in its use. Before initiating your beginning cardiolift, spend a couple of sessions in the gym getting instruction from floor personnel in the exercises and machines available in your facility. You should find all the basic machines and weights needed for the exercises illustrated in figure 4.5, which are easy to learn and will provide a comprehensive and balanced workout.

The first three resistance exercises shown in figure 4.5 exercise the muscles that operate the knee and hip joints. The lower body, along with the core or abdomen, is the foundation for all physical activity—walking, lifting, and playing sports. Unless your lower body and core are strong, you cannot do overhead presses or other upper body exercises nearly as well. These first three exercises will work the three main lower body joints—ankles, knees, and hips—and the full constellation of muscles around those joints, from toes to glutes.

Your cardiolift workout continues with the largest upper body muscles, including the back (figure 4.5, exercise 4), chest (exercise 5), and shoulders (exercise 6). Your arms are worked by most of the exercises shown. The sequence concludes with the core—the midsection of the body, including the abdomen (exercise

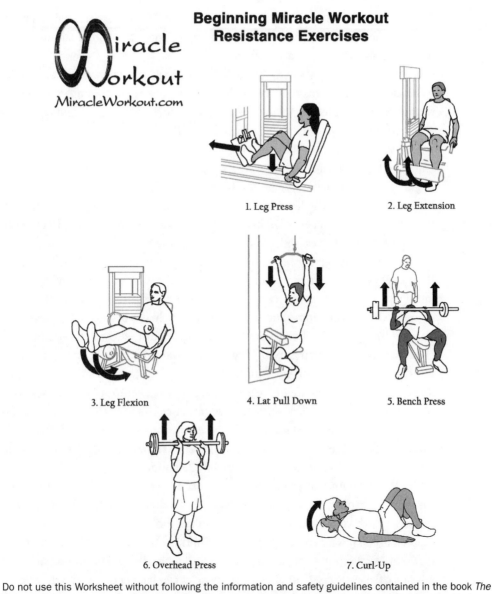

Beginning Miracle Workout Resistance Exercises

MiracleWorkout.com

1. Leg Press

2. Leg Extension

3. Leg Flexion

4. Lat Pull Down

5. Bench Press

6. Overhead Press

7. Curl-Up

FIGURE 4.5 **Beginning IBC Resistance Exercises** Here is a basic sequence of resistance, or weightlifting, exercises that target all of the major body muscles. Arrows show the direction, range, and trajectory or arc of the concentric phase of each movement. Always use a spotter for the bench press (exercise 5), unless you use a Smith Rack and safety stops. You can also do the overhead press (exercise 6) using a Smith Rack.

7), which acts as the primary support system for all other exercises and activities. The core includes your whole trunk, including not just the abdominal muscles in front, but also the spinal erectors in the lower back. The best exercises for the spinal erectors—bench squats, dead lifts, and back extensions—are also more technical and may increase the risk of lower back injury in beginning exercisers. If your gym has a seated back exercise (spinal erector) machine—a kind of reverse action from a seated abdominal curl machine—that is a good option to add to the sequence shown to complete working the core.

Note that the sequence of resistance exercises in figure 4.5 starts with the large leg muscles, works progressively toward smaller muscles, and finishes up with core exercises. The leg muscles are first in this sequence in part to help sustain your warm-up and elevated heart rate, while core exercise is done last to keep your abdominal muscles fresh to support each of the preceding exercises.

You are ready for the fully integrated third and final phase of the beginning IBC workout: the cardiolift. Here you alternate resistance exercises with cardio, following the pattern of the cardiorom phase. Copy figure 4.5, or print it from www.MiracleWorkout.com (click on "Exercises"), in 8½-by-11-inch format, and attach it to your workout clipboard for reference. Your first cardiolift session, like all of your workouts, starts with a big drink of water 20 minutes preceding your warm-up. After your warm-up, your heart rate will drop as you set up the leg press machine. Cardio-accelerate to raise your heart rate back into your moderate heart rate window, and do 8–12 repetitions of your first resistance exercise, the leg press (figure 4.5, exercise 1). Start with light weight—say, one-quarter of your body weight. If that's too heavy, back off a bit, and if it's too light, add some weight. Count the weight of the empty sled, typically 35 pounds.

Follow the same pattern for the remainder of your cardiolift workout—set up the weight machine, cardio-accelerate, do the exercise, put the weights away, wipe the bench with your sweat towel, take a drink whether or not you are thirsty, and proceed to the next exercise in figure 4.5. Continue this sequence until you reach the final exercise, abdominal crunches, and double the repetitions—that is, do 16–24 partial curl-ups. Your abdominal muscles can handle more repetitions than most other muscles of the body.

In this first cardiolift workout, you may already encounter the most common complication with IBC—access to motorized cardio machines for your intermittent cardio-acceleration. Many gyms get crowded during certain peak hours, and cardio machines are in special demand, so it can be a logistical challenge to maintain access to a cardio machine and a weight machine at the same time. You may encounter the same problem, on a smaller scale, during the cardiorom phase. The ideal solution would be a gym with a cardio machine next to every weight area or resistance machine—my dream gym—but unfortunately, most health clubs are not yet arranged this way.

Until then, here are some possible solutions:

- Exercise at slack hours, when the aerobic machines are less crowded.
- Learn all the cardio machines so you can switch as necessary during peak hours. Rotation among cardio machines is a good idea anyway, to reduce staleness and lower the risk of overtraining injuries.
- Talk to your gym manager about reserving some cardio machines for brief cardio-accelerations.
- Ask your gym manager to consider acquiring more cardio machines.
- Cardio-accelerate using nonmotorized options.

If you choose a nonmotorized option for cardio-acceleration, the most convenient place to do it is right next to the weight or machine you are about to use. That, however, can affect other exercisers in the immediate area. Discuss your cardio-acceleration plan, and options, with your gym manager and floor personnel, so that they understand and support your IBC workout. They may be able to help you make arrangements that will not bother other exercisers.

Once you're accustomed to the cardiolift, you will be able to complete the beginning version in about 20 minutes—1 minute per exercise for preceding cardio-acceleration, and 30 seconds each for the setup, exercise, and breakdown. Add to this the 5-minute warm-up, and you still have 5 minutes to do the ROM sequence (figure 4.4) as your cooldown, but in this case with no intermittent cardio-acceleration. That will bring to 30 minutes your workout time for the beginning cardiolift phase.* It's a 5–20–5 workout: 5 minutes for your warm-up, 20 minutes for resistance exercises interpolated with cardio-driving, and 5 minutes for your ROM cooldown.

Form Leads Function

In architecture, form often follows function, but in exercise, it's the other way around. Get the form right, and the function follows. Weightlifting form has three elements—support, movement, and breathing. Support means adopting a stable

---

* Warm-up, 5 minutes; resistance exercises, 13 minutes; intermittent cardio-acceleration bouts, 7 minutes; cooldown, 5 minutes; for a total workout time of about 30 minutes.

stance or position during every resistance exercise. For standing exercises, spread your feet to shoulder width, feet flat on the floor, knees slightly bent, and spine straight, looking straight ahead in the neutral position. This stance will keep your center of gravity within the support base established by your feet. For sitting exercises, keep your feet flat against surfaces, spine straight, and look ahead. For all resistance exercises, keep your head straight (the neutral spine position), stay alert, cultivate perfect symmetry, and stay safely clear of other exercisers.

The second element of form is movement. In resistance exercises, movement includes two phases: concentric and eccentric. Concentric movement occurs when the working muscle shortens during force application, as in the upward movement of a barbell during arm curls. Eccentric movements occur when the working muscle lengthens during force application, as in the downward movement of an arm curl. In the line drawings of resistance exercises (such as figure 4.5), the arrows point in the direction of the concentric movement. The concentric movement is no more important than the eccentric movement—on the contrary, the majority of muscle development may occur during the eccentric phase. Give equal time and attention to both the concentric and eccentric movement phase of every exercise. During the eccentric movement, brake the weight smoothly and evenly through the whole range of movement. A good rule of thumb at the beginning and intermediate level is to complete each movement—concentric and eccentric—in two full seconds.

Breathing correctly during resistance training is paramount, and may make a difference of 10–20 percent in exercise benefits. In the beginning IBC workout, complete one full breathing cycle for each exercise movement cycle (concentric–eccentric). Exhale completely during the concentric phase of every movement (arrows in figure 4.5), and inhale fully on the eccentric phase. For most people, the concentric phase feels like it takes the greatest exertion, so we can restate the breathing rule more simply: Exhale on exertion.

Correct breathing is important for both mental and physical reasons. It calms the mind and assists the circulation of blood. We usually think of the heart as the primary pump for our circulation, but during movement the rest of the muscles assist, perhaps equally with the heart. Your heart pumps the blood out to the body, but your muscles push blood back to your heart. Your breathing and movements during weightlifting must be synchronized properly to engage this supplemental heart. When you exhale on exertion, your internal chest pressure declines just when the contraction of your muscles is pushing blood back to your heart, enabling unobstructed venous return. Breathe wrong and you impede your heart, but exhale on exertion and your whole body becomes a heart.

Three Safety Tips for Weightlifting

Before you head down to the gym, here are three safety tips to reduce the risk of injury during weightlifting and therefore keep you exercising regularly. First, avoid heavy weights in the beginning, particularly for the leg press (figure 4.5, exercise 1) and leg extension (exercise 3), but also for the overhead press (exercise 6). Begin your resistance training program with an empty bar, sled, or rack—and work first on mastering form. As you become familiar with the exercises, you can add weight at your own rate to whatever poundage that requires strong effort and causes no more than weak pain.

Second, proper form is a key to lowering the risk of injury. When you do the leg press, for example, stay perfectly symmetrical—square in the chair—to avoid torque on the knees, hips, and pelvic girdle. The overhead press (figure 4.5, exercise 6) compresses and strengthens the backbone. Keep your spine straight ("neutral") to avoid excess translational stress on your lower (lumbar and sacral) vertebrae. With lighter weights, form is more forgiving, but when you advance to heavier weights later, and particularly at more advanced levels, incorrect form is a prime cause of injury. It's worth mastering form from the outset to reduce the risk. Particularly in the beginning stages, and periodically thereafter get feedback on your form from trained gym personnel in your health club.

Third, learn early to understand and respect the idiosyncrasies of each resistance exercise. The leg and overhead presses noted above, for example, require special attention. So does the leg extension exercise (figure 4.5, exercise 2), particularly for women (chapter 9). Open-chain leg extension done without weight does not compress the knee joint, enabling the shinbone (tibia) to translate forward relative to the thighbone (femur). All that keeps them together are the cruciate ligaments inside the knee. The exercise therefore stresses those ligaments, requiring care. The stress, however, is just what strengthens the cruciate ligaments and reduces the risk of knee injury. When you do the free-weight (barbell) bench press (figure 4.5, exercise 5), use a spotter as shown in the illustration to avoid dropping the bar on yourself. You can do without a spotter by performing the bench press using the Smith Rack, where the barbell moves vertically in fixed tracks. In that case, however, set the safety stops near the bottom of the tracks to prevent the bar from landing on you.

Use these safety tips to protect yourself and keep your exercise program rolling. Nothing sets your exercise program back like an injury, and it is worth the continual vigilance to lower the risk. Just keep in mind that exercising is far less risky than not exercising. As long as you are in good health and open to understanding your body, start with light weights, perfect your form, and advance using the IBC method of progression to optimize effort and minimize pain—you should be just fine. If you harbor any lingering doubts, consult your physician or personal trainer.

Workout Logs

Some people thrive on keeping exercise records, while others find it a bore. IBC offers the choice. Particularly at the beginning level, you can skip the workout logs and just get used to the workout. If you do want to keep simple records, you can record your progress on copies of your ROM and resistance exercise worksheets (figures 4.4 and 4.5). Keep track of the duration of ROM exercises, and/or the repetitions and/or weight that you will use in your next cardiolift session, beside the drawing of the corresponding exercise. The annotated forms then become a record of your progress.

There is reason, however, to keep more complete records. For one thing, workout records provide a chronicle of progress that can be highly motivating. There's nothing more encouraging than watching your heart, muscles, and joints strengthen measurably, week after week, for months. We've created the IBC workout logs in the appendix to this chapter to make record keeping as simple as possible. These forms have a space to record your cardiovascular data, the weight you lift during the cardiolift phase, your repetitions, and your responses to perceived exertion and perceived pain for each exercise. On that basis, you prescribe your next workout on the spot. When you next come to the gym, your path is clear. This process is an example of a motivational method called stimulus control, which we'll learn more about later (chapter 8). Instructions for using the logs are contained in the appendix, and the logs are available also in 8½-by-11-inch format from www.MiracleWorkout.com (click on "Workout Logs").

Maintain Your Gains

You have learned the three elements of IBC—integrate exercise, elevate heart rate during exercise, and progress based on biofeedback. This brings you to a choice point: Stand pat, or graduate. Stick with the beginning IBC program for now if it meets your exercise needs and goals. You can do the beginning cardiolift indefinitely, if you wish, and you will harvest many if not most of the benefits of exercise. If you are happy where you are, you have attained the fifth stage of exercise, maintenance (chapter 8). Your goal now is simply to hold on to the gains you have already realized.

Maintenance does not mean doing the same exercises indefinitely. That is a recipe for boredom, and risks overuse injury. Instead, maintenance requires varying exercises and type of exercise every few weeks or months, or cross-training, and variation over the year, or periodization. To cross-train, incorporate new aerobic exercises and new resistance exercises such as those introduced in chapters 5 and 6, or draw on new exercises from other sources. When you shift to other exercises that work the same muscle in different ways, you shock the muscle, use it more fully, and enhance its development naturally.* If you have a special physical interest or goal—toned upper arms, for example, or firm thighs, or well-defined abdominal muscles, or a flat tummy—now would be your opportunity to add exercises to develop these muscles or groups. You may want to consider a more complete core workout by learning and adding the dead lift. Especially if you are older, an athlete, or a golfer,† work those hips by adding hip abduction and adduction resistance exercises (chapter 5).

Periodize your IBC program over the year with seasonal variation. In a cold climate, winter can be a good time for an indoor workout, while spring, summer, and fall may support outdoor workouts. If summers are hot and humid where you live, that may be the season for the comfort and safety of a controlled gym environment, and the winters may be better for outdoor exercise. You can periodize your program by rotating seasonally among types of exercise—cardio, cardiorom, cardiolift—or even take a summer cardio sabbatical, during which you focus on recreational aerobics such as power walking, hiking, climbing, cycling, rowing, or swimming. It beats a conventional sedentary vacation.

However you elect to periodize your beginning IBC program, your main goal is to stay active across seasons and throughout the years. Your exercise must be fun and stay fun—if you love it, you will keep doing it for life, and that is the goal. If you do take a break, or suffer an exercise relapse (chapter 8), try at a minimum to keep your cardiovascular system in good enough shape to return comfortably to the beginning workout at the same level you left. That means getting the surgeon general's minimum of 30 minutes of moderate physical activity accumulated over the day, three to five days a week.

---

* When you shift from one exercise to another that uses the same muscles, you recruit new combinations of motor units—new individual nerve cells and the muscle fibers they innervate. The result is that you work previously unused fibers and regions of the same muscles, growing each muscle and muscle group to its full biological potential.

† Recent research has found a good correlation between hip strength and lower golf scores. For additional strengthening tips for golf (and other sports), see chapter 7.

Graduation

When you have completed the beginning IBC program described in this chapter and remained at that level for a while, revisit the goals of your exercise program in light of your learning and, especially, in view of your new body. If you are happy where you are, stay right there. You can use the beginning IBC workout for life, incorporating all the variations you will learn in chapter 7. On the other hand, you may decide that your goals now extend beyond health and wellness, to physical fitness. If that is the case, you are physically and mentally ready to graduate to the intermediate IBC program. The concepts and procedures you have learned in this chapter apply equally to the intermediate and advanced IBC programs. You are well along on the IBC learning curve, and the next chapter will carry you to that next level.

Appendix to Chapter 4

PAR-Q and Symptoms Questionnaire

The questionnaires in this appendix will help you determine whether it is safe for you to do the moderate exercise of the Beginning Miracle Workout. There are two forms. The first is the PAR-Q* form developed by the Canadian Society for Exercise Physiology. The second form is the Symptoms Questionnaire, based on recommendations by the American College of Sports Medicine.[†]

If you answered no to every question on both forms, the ACSM indicates that it is safe for you to do *moderate* exercise, as in the Beginning Miracle Workout, without a medical exam and without a doctor-supervised exercise test. If you answered yes to any question on either form, however, or if you expect to exercise at a *vigorous* level, complete the risk stratification questionnaire in chapter 5 and clarify the issue with your doctor before you change your physical activity. Talk to your doctor also if you are taking any medication, or if you have any old injuries or operations, to make sure they will not complicate your exercise program.

Instructions for Use of Beginning Miracle Workout Logs

There are two different forms contained in this appendix: the prescribed and the generic beginning Miracle Workout log. The prescribed workout log lists the seven resistance exercises shown in figure 4.5, while the generic workout log leaves the exercise spaces blank for you to write in whatever resistance exercises you choose. The instructions for using the beginning Miracle Workout log are the same for both the prescribed and generic workout logs.

Get familiar first with the general form of the log. Note that there are spaces at the top for personal information, followed by three boxes. Each box has columns for recording three workouts, distinguished by block shading. The first box at the top is for date and day; the second for recording your cardiolift data; and the third for recording overall workout parameters. Scan the headings of columns and rows in preparation for the instructions that follow. If you choose your own resistance exercise (generic log), put the abdominal core exercises last (exercise 7).

Start at the top by entering your name if you wish, followed by the upper limit of your heart rate window for active rest, your lower moderate heart rate training window limit, your upper limit, and your target (middle) moderate value. Calculate these values as percentages of your maximum heart rate (HR_{MAX} estimated by

---

* Source: Physical Activity Readiness Questionnaire (PAR-Q) © 2002. Reprinted with permission from the Canadian Society for Exercise Physiology. http://www.csep.ca/forms.asp.

† Source: American College of Sports Medicine. Reprinted with permission.

PAR-Q & YOU

(A Questionnaire for People Aged 15 to 69)

Regular physical activity is fun and healthy, and increasingly more people are starting to become more active every day. Being more active is very safe for most people. However, some people should check with their doctor before they start becoming much more physically active.

If you are planning to become much more physically active than you are now, start by answering the seven questions in the box below. If you are between the ages of 15 and 69, the PAR-Q will tell you if you should check with your doctor before you start. If you are over 69 years of age, and you are not used to being very active, check with your doctor.

Common sense is your best guide when you answer these questions. Please read the questions carefully and answer each one honestly: check YES or NO.

YES	NO		
☐	☐	1.	**Has your doctor ever said that you have a heart condition <u>and</u> that you should only do physical activity recommended by a doctor?**
☐	☐	2.	**Do you feel pain in your chest when you do physical activity?**
☐	☐	3.	**In the past month, have you had chest pain when you were not doing physical activity?**
☐	☐	4.	**Do you lose your balance because of dizziness or do you ever lose consciousness?**
☐	☐	5.	**Do you have a bone or joint problem (for example, back, knee or hip) that could be made worse by a change in your physical activity?**
☐	☐	6.	**Is your doctor currently prescribing drugs (for example, water pills) for your blood pressure or heart condition?**
☐	☐	7.	**Do you know of <u>any other reason</u> why you should not do physical activity?**

If you answered

YES to one or more questions

Talk with your doctor by phone or in person BEFORE you start becoming much more physically active or BEFORE you have a fitness appraisal. Tell your doctor about the PAR-Q and which questions you answered YES.

- You may be able to do any activity you want — as long as you start slowly and build up gradually. Or, you may need to restrict your activities to those which are safe for you. Talk with your doctor about the kinds of activities you wish to participate in and follow his/her advice.
- Find out which community programs are safe and helpful for you.

NO to all questions

If you answered NO honestly to <u>all</u> PAR-Q questions, you can be reasonably sure that you can:

- start becoming much more physically active — begin slowly and build up gradually. This is the safest and easiest way to go.
- take part in a fitness appraisal — this is an excellent way to determine your basic fitness so that you can plan the best way for you to live actively. It is also highly recommended that you have your blood pressure evaluated. If your reading is over 144/94, talk with your doctor before you start becoming much more physically active.

DELAY BECOMING MUCH MORE ACTIVE:

- if you are not feeling well because of a temporary illness such as a cold or a fever — wait until you feel better; or
- if you are or may be pregnant — talk to your doctor before you start becoming more active.

PLEASE NOTE: If your health changes so that you then answer YES to any of the above questions, tell your fitness or health professional. Ask whether you should change your physical activity plan.

<u>Informed Use of the PAR-Q</u>: The Canadian Society for Exercise Physiology, Health Canada, and their agents assume no liability for persons who undertake physical activity, and if in doubt after completing this questionnaire, consult your doctor prior to physical activity.

No changes permitted. You are encouraged to photocopy the PAR-Q but only if you use the entire form.

NOTE: If the PAR-Q is being given to a person before he or she participates in a physical activity program or a fitness appraisal, this section may be used for legal or administrative purposes.

"I have read, understood and completed this questionnaire. Any questions I had were answered to my full satisfaction."

NAME _____

SIGNATURE _____ DATE_____

SIGNATURE OF PARENT _____ WITNESS _____
or GUARDIAN (for participants under the age of majority)

> **Note: This physical activity clearance is valid for a maximum of 12 months from the date it is completed and becomes invalid if your condition changes so that you would answer YES to any of the seven questions.**

Source: Physical Activity Readiness Questionnaire (PAR-Q) © 2002. Reprinted with permission from the Canadian Society for Exercise Physiology. http://www.csep.ca/forms.asp.

SYMPTOMS QUESTIONNAIRE

Do you ever experience any of the following signs or symptoms?

Yes   No

☐   ☐   Pain, discomfort in the chest, neck, jaw, arms, or other areas

☐   ☐   Shortness of breath at rest or with mild exertion

☐   ☐   Dizziness or syncope (fainting)

☐   ☐   Difficulty breathing while lying down, or sudden awakening at night with difficulty breathing and/or anxiety

☐   ☐   Swelling of the ankles

☐   ☐   Heart arrhythmia of any kind (e.g., skipped or accelerated beats)

☐   ☐   Heart palpitations (unusually strong or rapid beats) or tachycardia (bouts of accelerated heart rate)

☐   ☐   Intermittent pain in any extremities (claudication)

☐   ☐   Heart murmur

☐   ☐   Unusual fatigue or shortness of breath with usual activities

☐   ☐   Asthma or other pulmonary diseases

☐   ☐   Diabetes or other metabolic diseases

A "yes" answer to any question on this questionnaire requires clarification with your physician before you begin any exercise program.

From the Guidelines of the American College of Sports Medicine, *ACSM's Guidelines for Exercise Testing and Prescription,* sixth edition. (Philadelphia: Lippincott Williams & Wilkins, 2000), box 2.1, p. 25. Copyright © 2000 by American College of Sports Medicine. Reproduced by permission of Lippincott Williams & Wilkins.

Beginning Miracle Workout Log, Cardiolift Phase, Prescribed

Name _____

CARDIOVASCULAR PARAMETERS AND HEART RATE TRAINING WINDOW

Active Rest _____ **BPM**   **Lower** _____ **BPM**   **Upper** _____ **BPM**   **Target** _____ **BPM**
(55 percent HR_{MAX})   (55 percent HR_{MAX})   (69 percent HR_{MAX})   (62 percent HR_{MAX})

WORKOUT# _____		WORKOUT# _____		WORKOUT# _____	
Date (m/d/y)	Day of Week	Date (m/d/y)	Day of Week	Date (m/d/y)	Day of Week

FREE WEIGHTS AND EXERCISE MACHINES

Exercise	Weight (lbs.)	Reps (8–12)	Pain > weak (Y/N)	Exert > strong (Y/N)	Weight (lbs)	Reps (8–12)	Pain > weak (Y/N)	Exert > strong (Y/N)	Weight (lbs)	Reps (8–12)	Pain > weak (Y/N)	Exert > strong (Y/N)
1. Leg Press												
2. Leg Extension												
3. Leg Flexion												
4. Lat Pull-Down												
5. Bench Press												
6. Overhead Press												
7. Core (Abdominals)												

OVERALL WORKOUT PARAMETERS

Weight Before/After	/	/	/
Water Used (liters)			
Observations and Comments			

Beginning Miracle Workout Log, Cardiolift Phase, Generic

Name _____

CARDIOVASCULAR PARAMETERS AND HEART RATE TRAINING WINDOW

Active Rest _____ **BPM**   **Lower** _____ **BPM**   **Upper** _____ **BPM**   **Target** _____ **BPM**

(55 percent HR_{MAX})   (55 percent HR_{MAX})   (69 percent HR_{MAX})   (62 percent HR_{MAX})

WORKOUT# _____		WORKOUT# _____		WORKOUT# _____	
Date (m/d/y)	**Day of Week**	**Date (m/d/y)**	**Day of Week**	**Date (m/d/y)**	**Day of Week**

FREE WEIGHTS AND EXERCISE MACHINES

Exercise (Write In)	Weight (lbs.)	Reps (8–12)	Pain > weak (Y/N)	Exert > strong (Y/N)	Weight (lbs)	Reps (8–12)	Pain > weak (Y/N)	Exert > strong (Y/N)	Weight (lbs)	Reps (8–12)	Pain > weak (Y/N)	Exert > strong (Y/N)
1.												
2.												
3.												
4.												
5.												
6.												
7.												

OVERALL WORKOUT PARAMETERS

Weight Before/After	/	/	/
Water Used (liters)			
Observations and Comments			

the formula, 220 minus your age in years), and use the percentages indicated in table 4.1 to find your heart rate values. Round all of your values to the nearest five to make them easier to remember, and check them against the decadal ranges in table 4.2 to confirm your calculations.

As you begin each workout, record the workout number, date, and day of the week in the top box. After a 5-minute warm-up, load the weights you will use for the leg press in your first workout (prescribed workout) or whatever exercise you choose to do first (generic workout). The empty sled (leg press machine) or bars (free weights) have a weight that should be counted in the weight you record. Record the weight you use for each exercise in the space provided in the box labeled FREE WEIGHTS AND EXERCISE MACHINES.

Then do a cardio-acceleration to elevate your heart rate into your moderate heart rate training window, followed by eight to twelve repetitions of the leg press (prescribed workout) or your first exercise (generic workout). Record the weight and repetitions you used in the two columns that follow the exercise. Immediately when you complete your set, record whether any pain you felt during the leg press was greater than *weak* (yes or no), and whether the exertion you felt was greater than *strong* (yes or no). If both answers were no, for your next workout increase the repetitions by one or two, or the weight by 5 or 10 pounds, and record the new values immediately in the corresponding space for your next workout. As a rule, progress in 5-pound increments for small-muscle groups (generally upper body), and 10-pound increments for large-muscle groups (generally lower body). Each time you advance in weight or repetitions, circle the corresponding number. That rewards your advance, and enables you to tell at a glance how many advances you are achieving over time, which is the most immediate measure of your progression. When you advance to twelve repetitions and are ready to progress further, reduce the repetitions back to eight and increase the weight by 5 or 10 pounds.

If you answered yes to the question about perceived pain, record the same weight and repetitions for your next workout, and seek professional assistance to understand the cause of the pain before you continue or work out again. If you answered yes to the question about perceived exertion, record the same weight and repetitions for your next workout. You have just implemented the IBC method of progression, which will keep you advancing in comfort as fast as your genes will permit and with minimum risk of injury.

Move to the next exercise—either the leg extension machine (prescribed workout) or whatever exercise you choose (generic workout), and set or load your weight. Do another cardio-acceleration, and then perform the indicated repetitions while your heart rate is elevated. Again record your answers to the pain and exertion questions, and progress as with the first exercise. Increment the weight by 5 or 10 pounds, or raise the repetitions by one or two.

When you are finished with the resistance exercises, do a 5-minute cooldown using the ROM exercises shown in figure 4.4. Keep your heart rate near the upper boundary of moderate exercise, 55 percent of your HR_{MAX}, while you cool down. Then record your OVERALL WORKOUT PARAMETERS in the bottom box. Record your body weight before and after your workout; if it is the same, you drank enough water. Next, record the amount of water you drank during the workout, to help you dial in your correct hydration volume. The final row, labeled OBSERVATIONS AND COMMENTS, provides a space for recording any other relevant information, including general impressions of your physical or emotional state following your workout. Use this box also to footnote and describe details of any pain you experienced during individual resistance exercises. Study your recorded observations and comments over time to detect repetitive or persistent pain, or any other pattern that may merit attention.

5

Your Intermediate Miracle Workout

The intermediate IBC program is for you if you are in good health, already an exerciser, have worked out continuously for the past few months, and are in good physical shape, such as when you have recently completed the beginning IBC program. The goals at the intermediate level include all the health and wellness benefits of the beginning level, but extend further to full physical fitness. Controlling weight and feeling good remain central, as do maintaining a high level of energy and managing everyday pain. In addition, the intermediate IBC program will sculpt your body. You may seek toned and shaped muscles, or washboard abs, or bulging biceps—but at this point, you are not yet too concerned with peak athletic performance, the province of the advanced IBC program.

There is an easy way to tell whether you are ready to start the intermediate program. You should be able to exercise continuously at moderate intensity for at least half an hour in comfort—a moment you'll reach when you have done the beginning cardiolift for a while. You also need to know the basic form of the IBC workout, which you can get by doing the beginning level described in the preceding chapter. This chapter assumes you know about hydration, exercise form, and the safety tips and idiosyncrasies of individual resistance exercises as described in the preceding chapter.

The most noticeable difference at the intermediate level is workout intensity. Attaining physical fitness requires that you exercise vigorously, rather than moderately, an hour per workout three days a week. The intermediate workout takes a greater commitment, and delivers greater rewards. If you are a weight watcher or want to lose additional pounds, for example, you have arrived. Abundant research demonstrates that a bout of vigorous exercise revs up your metabolism for hours, and accelerates fat burning in particular. If you're ready to sweat—and if you want to feel exhilarated the way nature intended—you are the ideal candidate for the intermediate IBC program. If you think the intermediate workout will take more energy than you have, see the accompanying sidebar.

Play It Safe

The heart of an average person pumps 15 liters of blood every minute at rest—that's about 1,000 quarts per hour. Moderate exercise, such as in the beginning IBC program, approximately doubles this flow. Vigorous exercise, as in the intermediate program, increases blood flow by four to eight times, to as much as 8,000 quarts per hour. It is essential to make sure your heart can handle that load before you start IBC at the intermediate level. Part of the process involves applying the risk assessment guidelines of the American College of Sports Medicine (ACSM). Start with the same two questionnaires described in the preceding chapter. Then go through the risk stratification procedure of the ACSM shown in the appendix to this chapter or online at www.MiracleWorkout.com (click on "Safety/Intermediate"). These procedures determine your cardiovascular risk category (low, moderate, high), which tells you whether you need a medical exam and a doctor-supervised exercise test before doing vigorous exercise. In this process of risk stratification, you also determine your weight category and the associated risk, if any, using the procedure described in the appendix or the Body Mass Index Calculator (www. MiracleWorkout.com; click on "BMI Calculator").

The Blueprint for Your Intermediate IBC Program

The intermediate IBC program follows the same pattern as the beginning program. The main differences are the intensity of exercise (vigorous instead of moderate), time (60 minutes instead of 30), and workload (more exercises and sets). Follow the blueprint in figure 5.1. Complete the same two preparatory steps described for the beginning IBC program—cardio and cardiorom—before your transition into the fully integrated cardiolift stage. That will strengthen your heart and joints incrementally at your own pace, based on your current capacities and goals.

When you can do vigorous cardiovascular exercise comfortably for 40 minutes, integrate Range of Motion (ROM) and then resistance exercises into your car-

Myth Buster 5: Exercise Is Too Hard

THE MYTH: Exercise takes too much energy. I'm already exhausted by the end of the day—how can I possibly add more?

As you move from the beginning to the intermediate level of IBC, you invest more energy. Perhaps you are concerned that it will simply take too much, draining your limited reserves. IBC does take energy, more than any conventional workout in a comparable time, and particularly as you move from the beginning to the intermediate level. At intermediate and advanced levels, you may even feel the need for a nap after the first few workouts, so indulge yourself if possible, or get extra sleep at night.

After a few workouts, however, your energy systems ignite in earnest. By that point, IBC will actually be giving you more energy than it takes. Many people who do IBC, particularly if they're deconditioned initially, note first the enormous new vitality it confers. You feel more energetic not only during workouts, but also between them. The net result—you have more energy not only to exercise, but also to bring to bear on everyday life and its activities.

How can you invest more energy in IBC, yet feel more energized? The answer lies in energy systems conditioning. Your three energy systems—first, second, and third gears (chapter 2)—respond to exercise just as dramatically as your muscles and heart, ligaments, and lungs. As they develop, these energy systems speed up their base rates, which not only is invigorating but also burns more calories every moment of the day and night.

Perhaps the greatest advantage of IBC for recreational exercisers and athletes alike is that it ignites your energy systems like no other workout. It is an energy systems training program. Far from feeling drained, once you establish your IBC program and stay with it for a few weeks, you will feel far more energized than before you started, and perhaps more energized than you imagined possible.

THE REALITY: IBC takes energy, but it gives back more by accelerating and tuning your three energy systems naturally.

The IBC Myth Buster

MYTH: Exercise takes too much energy.

FACT: IBC gives you far more energy than it takes.

dio routine. Then we will discuss how to maintain your fitness gains and, if you choose, to use your higher level of conditioning as a springboard to the advanced workout in the next chapter.*

FIGURE 5.1
THE THREE-STEP INTERMEDIATE IBC PROGRAM MADE SIMPLE

1. **Prerequisites.** Good physical condition, low cardiovascular risk category (see appendix, or go to www.MiracleWorkout.com and click on "Safety" and then "Intermediate"), or medical clearance.
2. **Intensity.** Vigorous exercise.
3. **Description.** Three steps: two preparatory and one integrated.

Step 1: Cardio (preparatory)

1. **Goal.** 40 minutes of vigorous cardio exercise in complete comfort.
2. **Method.** Self-paced, progressive aerobic (cardio) exercise.
3. **Time.** 40 minutes per workout, three workouts per week, for two to four weeks.

Step 2: Cardiorom (preparatory, partially integrated)

1. **Goal.** Integration of ROM with vigorous cardio exercise.
2. **Method.** Alternate vigorous cardio and ROM exercise.
3. **Time.** 50 minutes per workout, three workouts per week, for two to four weeks.

Step 3: Cardiolift (fully integrated)

1. **Goal.** Integration of weightlifting with vigorous cardio exercise followed by ROM cooldown.
2. **Method.** Alternate cardio and weightlifting exercise with a terminal ROM cooldown.
3. **Time.** 60 minutes per workout, three workouts per week, until maintenance stage or graduation to the advanced level.

The Intermediate Cardio Workout

The cardio phase of the intermediate IBC program starts with vigorous cardio exercise, corresponding to a heart rate of 70–89 percent of your maximum (table

---

* You can do a transitional workout, between beginning and intermediate, by doing the intermediate workout as described in this chapter but keeping your heart rate in the "moderate" rather than "vigorous" heart rate training window.

4.1). Determine your heart rate training window following the methodology in chapter 4, and confirm that your calculations are consistent with the decadal age values compiled in table 5.1.

Like the beginning IBC workout, you can do the intermediate workout anywhere you like (chapter 7). This chapter continues to describe the gym workout for consistency. Your goal in the cardio stage of the intermediate workout is to reach 40 continuous minutes of aerobic exercise with complete comfort—that is, with a Rating of Perceived Exertion (RPE) no greater than *strong,* and a Rating of Perceived Pain (RPP) no greater than *weak.*

TABLE 5.1
VIGOROUS EXERCISE HEART RATE TRAINING WINDOWS FOR DIFFERENT AGES BASED ON THE MAXIMUM HEART RATE METHOD

Age (years)	Maximum Heart Rate (220 – age)	Vigorous Heart Rate Training Window (BPM)
10	210	145–185
20	200	140–180
30	190	135–170
40	180	125–160
50	170	120–150
60	160	110–140
70	150	105–135
80	140	100–125
90	130	90–115
100	120	85–105

BPM = Beats per Minute. All ranges are rounded to the nearest five to make them easier to remember. The ranges shown assume you are not taking medications or substances that may influence heart rate up or down. If in doubt, consult with your doctor.

Hydrate early and often, starting with a large drink 20 minutes before your workout. Your heart monitor is strapped on, you know how to use it, and you know your heart rate training window. You have your water bottle and sweat towel in hand. As in the beginning cardio phase, consider this first intermediate cardio workout a practice session. Stay in your cardiovascular training window for just 5 or 10 minutes to get the feeling of vigorous exercise, collect biofeedback, and confirm your physical condition.

When you complete your first intermediate cardio session, remain active for the next few minutes. Stand, walk, or do light stretching and bending during this cooldown period, and gradually bring your heart rate down to the "active rest" level—around 55 percent of your maximum heart rate, the lower boundary of moderate exercise intensity (tables 4.1 and 4.2). The purpose of the cooldown is similar to the purpose of correct breathing during exercise—it facilitates venous return. If you stop exercise too abruptly, you may feel faint or dizzy. That's because your muscles no longer push blood back to your heart as fast as your heart can pump it out, and the impeded venous return can reduce blood supply to the head. If you feel faint, lower your head between your knees until the spell passes,* and seek assistance if it doesn't pass quickly.

The rule for progression at the intermediate level is the same as at the beginning level. At the end of your cardio workout, rate your perceived exertion and perceived pain using the Borg scale shown in figure 4.2. Add five minutes to the duration of your cardio workout every time you complete a session with a Rating of Perceived Exertion (RPE) no greater than *strong* and a Rating of Perceived Pain (RPP) no greater than *weak*. If you feel any pain greater than *weak*, identify the cause before you continue or progress. Repeat any cardio workout that you rate as harder than *strong* or more painful than *weak*. Don't be concerned about repeats—you'll grow into higher levels quickly.

How long it takes you to reach the 40-minute milestone of continuous vigorous aerobic exercise in full comfort depends on you—your initial physical condition, how motivated you are, and how often you exercise. Most people who start out in good shape require no more than four weeks. Take your time so your joints, ligaments, muscles, and heart can develop together at their own pace to minimize the risk of injury. Your purpose is to bring your whole body system up to the same level at the same rate, so each part can help and support every other part along the way.

* Placing your head between your knees lowers your heart rate abruptly. That's because your heart's first priority is to keep your head supplied with blood. When you lower your head between your knees, your head is now below your heart, and the blood flows downhill to your brain. Your heart therefore does not have to beat as fast to supply your head with enough blood.

The Intermediate Cardiorom Workout

Once you reach the 40-minute milestone, move to the intermediate cardiorom workout by integrating Range of Motion exercises into your cardio routine. Alternate cardio-acceleration bouts with ROM exercises, just as you did in the beginning cardiorom (chapter 4). The main purposes of the intermediate cardiorom stage are to learn the additional ROM exercises, increase your body flexibility, and strengthen your heart further in preparation for the cardiolift phase.

Because you have more time, you can expand your ROM sequence by three exercises (figure 5.2). The 12 ROM exercises in figure 5.2 engage every primary joint (the shoulders and hips), secondary joint (the knees and elbows), and add the tertiary joints (the wrists and ankles). There are hundreds of different ROM exercises available, however, any of which you can work into your cardiorom routine according to your specific interests and goals. There are even ROM exercises for the fingers, toes, and tongue! Get creative if you want; choose from the many good books on the topic. Bob and Jean Anderson's *Stretching* is a popular standard. Alternatively, take a ROM course through your health club, or learn additional ROM exercises from a personal trainer. If you select a different sequence of ROM exercises from those shown here, make sure they are comprehensive and balanced across muscles, joints, and the whole body.

After selecting your ROM exercises, integrate them with cardiovascular exercise. Copy figure 5.2 or download it in 8½-by-11-inch format from www.Miracle-Workout.com (click on "Exercises"), and attach it to a clipboard to prop up in your ROM exercise area. Warm up with vigorous cardio exercise for 10 minutes, and then alternate short, intense cardio-acceleration bouts with each ROM exercise. In your first cardiorom session, hold each ROM position for 15 seconds. As you become more flexible over the next couple of weeks, gradually increase your hold time to 30 or more seconds. You should complete your ROM sequence in less than 40 minutes, including the intermittent cardio-acceleration bouts. Taking into account the time for your warm-up, you will have a few minutes left for your active cooldown. Stay active for at least 5 minutes at 55 percent of your maximum heart rate ("active rest") for your cooldown. Your workout time for the intermediate cardiorom workout should be around 50 minutes.*

As in the beginning cardiorom, you will discover during the intermediate workout that your heart rate drops during each ROM exercise because ROM takes

---

* Ten minutes for your warm-up, twelve 1-minute intermittent cardio-driving bouts, twelve ROM exercises at less than 1 minute each, 5 minutes of "transaction" time, and a 5-minute cooldown, for a total workout time of a little under 50 minutes.

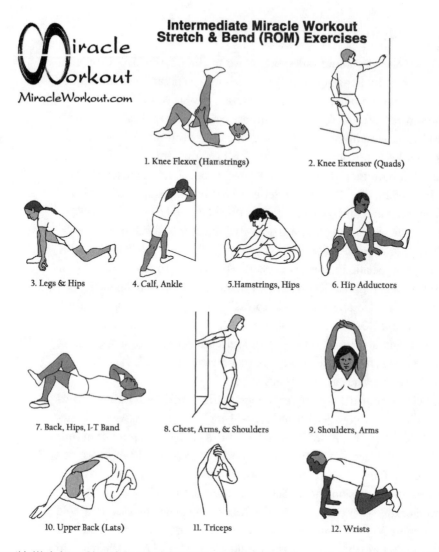

Intermediate Miracle Workout Stretch & Bend (ROM) Exercises

MiracleWorkout.com

1. Knee Flexor (Hamstrings)

2. Knee Extensor (Quads)

3. Legs & Hips

4. Calf, Ankle

5. Hamstrings, Hips

6. Hip Adductors

7. Back, Hips, I-T Band

8. Chest, Arms, & Shoulders

9. Shoulders, Arms

10. Upper Back (Lats)

11. Triceps

12. Wrists

Do not use this Worksheet without following the information and safety guidelines contained in the book *The Miracle Workout*. The Miracle Workout, and its agents, assume no liability for persons who use this Worksheet or change their exercise or physical activity. Copyright © 2004 by W. Jackson Davis. This Worksheet may be reproduced for personal use only.

FIGURE 5.2 **Intermediate IBC Stretch & Bend (ROM) Exercises** Here is a good intermediate sequence of Range of Motion exercises that adds to the beginning sequence shown in figure 4 of chapter 4. Three new ROM exercises are added, for calf and ankle (exercise 4), hamstrings and hips (exercise 5), and wrists and forearms (exercise 12). As in beginning ROM exercises, hold each static position shown for 15–30 seconds, and for unilateral exercises (all but exercises 6, 8, 9, and 12), stretch both sides of the body. Warm up before stretching and bending to minimize the risk of injury.

less effort than cardio. As your aerobic capacity increases with exercise, your heart rate will also recover faster after each cardio-acceleration. That's a good sign, because rapid heart rate recovery indicates better cardiovascular health and higher levels of aerobic fitness. Faster heart rate recovery does influence your workout, however, because as you get in better shape, it is increasingly harder to keep your heart rate elevated into your vigorous training window during each ROM exercise. Use one or more of these strategies to keep your heart rate elevated:

- Increase the intensity of your warm-up by working higher in your vigorous heart rate training window. If you are 20 years old and your window is 140–180 BPM, for example (table 5.1), warm up at 160 or 170 BPM instead of 140. More intense aerobic exercise pre-fatigues your cardiovascular system better, keeping your heart rate from recovering so fast during subsequent ROM exercises.
- Increase the duration of your warm-up, which also pre-fatigues your heart more.
- Increase the intensity of your cardio-acceleration bouts, giving your heart rate farther to fall during the subsequent ROM exercise and giving you more time to complete it without dropping out of your heart rate training window.

Progress through the intermediate cardiorom phase just as you did in the beginning cardiorom. Increase your workload whenever your RPE is *strong* or less and your RPP is *weak* or less. Raise your workload by increasing the intensity or the duration of your initial warm-up or the intermittent cardio-acceleration bouts between ROM exercises, and by incrementing the hold time of each ROM exercise to 30 seconds or longer. Move to the cardiolift phase of the intermediate IBC program when you can do a full cardiorom session—50 minutes in your vigorous heart rate training window—with an RPE of *strong* or less and an RPP of *weak* or less. It typically takes two to four weeks of regular workouts for most healthy, well-conditioned people to reach this milestone, but take as long as you need to make sure you're ready for the transition to the cardiolift phase.

The Intermediate Cardiolift Workout

This fully integrated workout blends resistance exercises into your cardio workout, just as did the beginning cardiolift (chapter 4), and concludes with a ROM cooldown. The main differences from the beginning level are the longer total time for resistance exercise and the greater intensity of your workout. The greater intensity comes from working in your vigorous rather than moderate heart rate target window, adding more resistance exercises, and doing two sets of each resistance exercise rather than one. You can do a transitional workout by performing one rather than two sets of each resistance exercise in your vigorous heart rate training window.

The purposes of the intermediate cardiolift are much the same as at the beginning level—you will learn additional resistance exercises, increase your overall body strength far above what was possible at the beginning level, and continue the accelerated strengthening of your cardiovascular system. The additional time (60 rather than 30 minutes) gives you room to add new resistance exercises, but the concept is identical—elevate your heart rate into the appropriate heart rate target window, using the cardio exercise that suits you best, and keep it there while you lift weights.

Figure 5.3 shows a sequence of resistance exercises that includes the seven basic exercises of the beginning IBC program and an additional two—arm curls (figure 5.3, exercise 7) and triceps extensions (exercise 8). Since you have more time at the intermediate level, you can begin to customize your workout with additional exercises such as those in figure 5.4. Mix and match to achieve specialized goals. Consider adding hip flexion and extension (figure 5.4, exercises 1 and 2), to strengthen your lower body foundation, or hip abduction/adduction (exercises 3 and 4). Or add shoulder shrugs (exercise 5) to strengthen your trapezius muscles. For wide, defined shoulders, work the front, middle, and rear deltoids (exercises 6–8). If you want shapely arms, add hammer curls or overhead triceps extensions (not shown). There are literally hundreds of different resistance exercises to choose from, depending on your specific interests.

You'll be able to complete two sets of nine resistance exercises that work the full body in the 40-minute target time for resistance training. An alternate approach is to work different regions or parts of the body on different days—alternate the upper and lower body in successive workouts, for example, or work the core one day and the rest the next day. If you use such split sessions, or if you design your own custom workout, retain balance across joints, muscles, and the whole body. Balance across joints and muscles should be incorporated into every workout, while balance across the whole body can be spread across longer periods, such as the entire workout week.

Once you select your intermediate resistance exercises and master form (support, movement, breathing; see chapter 4), you are ready to integrate them with cardio and ROM for the fully integrated intermediate cardiolift. Copy figures 5.3 and 5.4 from the following pages, or print them in 8½-by-11-inch format from www. MiracleWorkout.com (click on "Exercises"), and attach them to your workout clipboard. Then do a 10-minute warm-up with cardio exercise and start your integrated cardiolift.

Set up your first resistance exercise, the leg press (figure 5.3, exercise 1). The

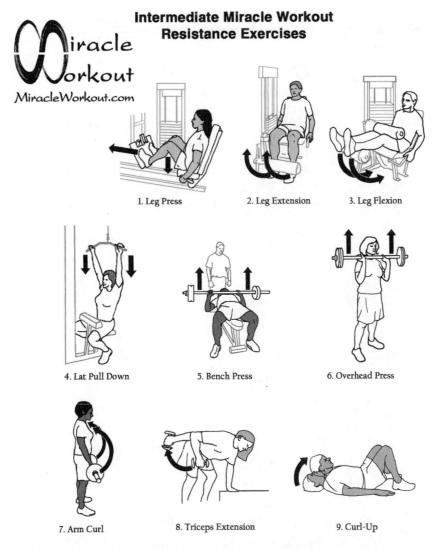

**Intermediate Miracle Workout
Resistance Exercises**

Miracle Workout
MiracleWorkout.com

1. Leg Press

2. Leg Extension

3. Leg Flexion

4. Lat Pull Down

5. Bench Press

6. Overhead Press

7. Arm Curl

8. Triceps Extension

9. Curl-Up

Do not use this Worksheet without following the information and safety guidelines contained in the book *The Miracle Workout*. The Miracle Workout, and its agents, assume no liability for persons who use this Worksheet or change their exercise or physical activity. Copyright © 2004 by W. Jackson Davis. This Worksheet may be reproduced for personal use only.

Figure 5.3 **Intermediate IBC Resistance Exercises** Here is an intermediate sequence of resistance exercises that extends the beginning sequence shown in figure 4.5. Added are specific weightlifting exercises for the biceps (exercise 7) and the opposing or antagonistic muscles, the triceps (exercise 8). Arrows show the direction, range, and trajectory or arc of the concentric phase of each movement. See the safety tips for certain of these exercises in chapter 4.

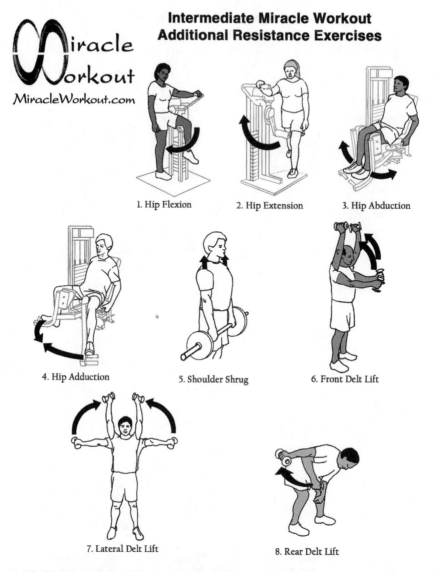

**Intermediate Miracle Workout
Additional Resistance Exercises**

Miracle Workout
MiracleWorkout.com

1. Hip Flexion   2. Hip Extension   3. Hip Abduction

4. Hip Adduction   5. Shoulder Shrug   6. Front Delt Lift

7. Lateral Delt Lift   8. Rear Delt Lift

FIGURE 5.4 **Additional Intermediate IBC Resistance Exercises** Here are some additional resistance or weightlifting exercises you can use to supplement the sequence shown in figure 5.3. Additional exercises shown here work the all-important hips (exercises 1–4) and shoulders (exercises 5–8). Arrows again show the direction, range, and trajectory or arc of the concentric phase of each exercise.

weightlifting safety tips in chapter 4 become especially important as you move to the heavier overloads of the intermediate cardiolift. Load your weight, spread your sweat towel on the bench, and prop your clipboard and water bottle nearby. Your heart rate will probably have dropped out of your vigorous training window, so elevate it with a short cardio-acceleration. Then, with your heart rate in the middle of your vigorous training window, do the leg press. Use a weight that lets you do 8–12 repetitions comfortably. After your first set of leg presses, cardio-accelerate again and then, unlike the beginning cardiolift, do a second set of the same leg press exercise using the same number of repetitions. Two sets of resistance exercises yield greater strength and endurance gains than a single set.

Replace your leg press weights, wipe the bench with your sweat towel, take a drink, and move to your second exercise station for the leg extension (figure 5.3, exercise 2). Do two sets of leg extensions at 8–12 repetitions, each preceded by cardio-acceleration, and move to your third resistance exercise. Continue this pattern to the end of your intermediate cardiolift session, doubling the repetitions for core exercises. You may feel the runner's high by the end of your warm-up, about 20 minutes into vigorous aerobic activity, and throughout the cardiolift phase. Make sure both sides of your body get equal time in the vigorous heart rate training window during unilateral exercises. You should be able to finish the entire resistance training segment of the intermediate cardiolift workout in about 40 minutes.*

The amount of weight and number of repetitions you use depend on your initial physical condition and on your exercise goals (table 5.2). If you seek definition and endurance, the conventional wisdom is to use higher numbers of repetitions (up to 20), with lighter weights (from half to two-thirds of your maximum lift; table 5.2). If you seek strength and power, use fewer repetitions and heavier weights—less than six repetitions per set, and up to 85 percent of your maximum lift.

The threshold weight usually recommended for most people for muscle adaptation, or growth in strength, is 65 percent of your one-repetition maximum (1-RM). A recent review of 140 different studies on weights and repetitions concluded that the optimum exercise dosage differs, however, for untrained and trained exercisers. According to this review, untrained people get stronger fastest when using 60 percent of their 1-RM values and work out three times per week, while trained people do better with 80 percent of their 1-RM and two workouts per week. Also according to this review, both untrained and trained individuals do best with four

---

* Based on 4.5 minutes per resistance exercise times nine exercises, assuming 30 seconds for setup, 60 seconds for cardio-acceleration, 45 seconds to perform the first set, 60 seconds for the next cardio-acceleration, 45 seconds to do the second set, and 30 seconds for disassembly and wipe-down.

TABLE 5.2
RELATION AMONG GOALS, REPETITIONS, LOAD, AND NUMBER OF SETS

Training Goal	Repetitions	% 1-RM	Perception of Weight	Number of Sets
Strength	<6	85	very heavy	2–6
Power (single-effort event)	1–2	80–90	heavy	3–5
Power (multi-effort event)	3–5	75–85	medium	3–5
Hypertrophy (bulk/definition)	6–12	67–85	medium	3–6
Endurance/definition	12–20	<67	light	3–6

From the National Strength and Conditioning Association (edited by T. R. Baechle and R. W. Earle), *Essentials of Strength Training and Conditioning,* second edition, p. 414, table 18.9. Copyright © 2000 by the National Strength and Conditioning Association. Adapted with permission from Human Kinetics (Champaign, IL).

sets of repetitions. If you don't know your 1-RM, start low with a comfortable weight and adjust upward, adjusting your weights and repetitions according to your specific exercise goals (table 5.2).

Your intermediate cardiolift has so far taken around 50 minutes, leaving 10 minutes for your cooldown. Do the same ROM sequence you did during cardiorom (30 seconds per stretch)—without, however, interpolating cardio exercise—to cool down. That will bring your heart rate down gradually to your active rest heart rate of around 55 percent of your maximum heart rate and still provide the benefits of ROM exercise. Your complete intermediate cardiolift workout therefore took 60 minutes.*

Your intermediate IBC cardiolift is a 10–40–10 program: 10 minutes of warm-up, 40 minutes for resistance training, and 10 minutes for your ROM cooldown.

---

* Warm-up, 10 minutes; resistance exercises, including intermittent cardio-acceleration, 40 minutes; ROM cooldown, 10 minutes; for a total workout time of 60 minutes.

The Full-Body Flush

One of the most rewarding aspects of the intermediate IBC workout is your sweat response. It will start about 15 or 20 minutes into your workout, about the same time the runner's high kicks in. By the time you finish 60 minutes of vigorous exercise, you will hopefully be good and soaked in perspiration. If you like, wear a sweatshirt to encourage the response—but be conscious of temperature regulation (chapter 9). The result—at the end of your workout you will feel vibrantly alive.

Some credit for this invigorated feeling may belong in part to the full-body flush. Up to two-thirds of the human body is water, and the average human body has about 8 quarts of blood. An intense IBC workout can replace as much as one-third of your total blood volume. IBC wrings large volumes of water from your body, carrying wastes and toxins with it. The full-body flush bathes you from the inside out, a natural cleansing that is unattainable in any other way. That's partly why it is important to drink pure, nonchlorinated water during an IBC workout. The full-body flush may be one of the most important health benefits of the intermediate IBC workout and its heightened sweat response.

Double Breathing

Breathing properly is a critical aspect of exercise (chapter 4). At the moderate-intensity exercise of the beginning level, you can easily complete one full breathing cycle in one full weightlifting movement cycle, exhaling completely during the two-second concentric movement (exhaling on exertion) and inhaling completely during the two-second eccentric movement. During the more vigorous intermediate workout, you may need to breathe faster yet still sustain the timing of your movements.

The solution is double breathing. Take two complete breaths during each single weightlifting movement cycle, rather than one. Inhale rapidly and completely during the pause at the end of each movement, concentric and eccentric, and exhale more slowly and completely during the movements themselves. That way you get two full breaths per weightlifting movement cycle, which you need, yet still exhale on every exertion, facilitating venous return. Double breathing keeps these two elements of form, movement and breathing, synchronized during vigorous exercise, sustaining the pumping function of your supplemental heart.

Progression and Gating

The IBC method of progression is partly what powers the incredible growth rates you can achieve. At the intermediate level, progression works the same as at the beginning level. After the second set of each resistance exercise, evaluate your RPE and RPP, record them on your workout log (appendix), and prescribe the weight and repetitions for the same resistance exercise in your next workout using that biofeedback.

The intermediate IBC workout adds a new wrinkle to the progression, however: gating. At the end of your workout, evaluate the RPE and RPP associated with the entire workout. If it took more than *strong* effort, or you felt overall pain greater than *weak,* repeat that workout next time—in other words, don't allow the advances you recorded for individual resistance exercises. The prolonged vigorous exercise of the intermediate IBC workout has a greater cumulative impact on your physiology, which can carry you closer to your physiological limit. Gating individual advances according to your overall workout evaluation keeps you exercising within a safe and enjoyable overall envelope as you progress in to the uncharted territory of steadily higher levels of intensity and workload.

If you are not the record-keeping type, or if your goals don't include rapid progression, skip the workout logs, or write down pertinent values on printouts of your ROM and resistance exercises. You may find workout records more necessary, however, in the intermediate IBC program, particularly as you reach higher levels. Workout logs tailored to the intermediate workout appear in the appendix to this chapter, along with instructions on their use; they're also downloadable from www.MiracleWorkout.com (click on "Workout Logs").

How to Avoid Overtraining

The intermediate IBC program exposes you increasingly to a new risk that can catch new exercisers by surprise—overtraining. IBC is so much fun that you may be tempted to overdo it, and time in the zone can get addictive. The irony of overtraining is that the most motivated exercisers are typically also the most vulnerable, including athletes in mid- or late season. Overuse injuries have pernicious multiplier effects. The body unconsciously compensates for the pain of an overtraining injury with subtle and unconscious shifts in movement and posture, placing greater and unnatural stress on other body parts. That imbalance can cause new complications and injuries.

You can recognize overtraining from four interrelated warning signs—the four P's: performance, physical, physiological, and psychological symptoms.

1. Performance symptoms of overtraining.
    The main indicator is burnout. You will know it if you have trouble recovering from vigorous exercise and your performance and motivation start to

deteriorate accordingly. Persistent fatigue, sluggishness, inconsistent performance, and long recovery times are also warning signs.

2. **Physical symptoms of overtraining.**

   Persistent minor pains, particularly at joints, tendons, or ligaments, are telltale signs. Treat such an overuse injury by modifying your exercise program. If you are using the treadmill for cardio work and your knees begin to ache from impact overuse, for example, first try switching to the elliptical trainer, or the cycle, or the rowing machine. If you develop an overuse injury from weight training, first try a different exercise using the same muscle groups. If the pain doesn't disappear, or worsens, give it a rest.

3. **Physiological symptoms of overtraining.**

   The surest physiological indicator is an elevated heart rate on awakening—10–20 percent higher than usual. An elevated pulse is also a sign of other medical conditions, however, so if your heart rate doesn't decline soon with rest, or if it's accompanied by other symptoms, see your doctor. Additional physiological symptoms of overtraining include cessation of menstruation, insomnia, loss of appetite, frequent bowel irregularities, and repeated upper respiratory tract infections from a fatigued immune system.

4. **Psychological symptoms of overtraining.**

   The mind–body connection works two ways—train right, and the mind and body stay in synchrony, but overtraining can result in general apathy, depression, decreased self-esteem, mood change, difficulty concentrating, and loss of competitive drive. If these symptoms arise, shift to maintenance mode (see next page), try a different routine such as the outdoor IBC workouts (chapter 7), or take a rest for a week or longer as required.

Resist any temptation to tough out, or work through, an overtraining injury. It generally doesn't work, and could set back your exercise program even further. Resist also any temptation to suppress the pain from an overtraining injury with drugs and then exercise. You may feel less pain, but the cause is still there, and continued exercise will just make it worse. Nature conferred on us the capacity to sense pain for a reason—to warn of impending or actual injury—and disguising the pain artificially may mute a voice we need to hear.

There is ultimately only one solution to overtraining: rest. Complete recovery from severe overtraining can take as long as weeks or even months. If you are an athlete in a key period of your sport season and you simply can't rest properly, try modifying and tapering. That is, reduce your training volume and intensity, and increase your carbohydrate intake (carbo-load), for three to seven days before a major competition. That will help give your body an opportunity to recover. Over-training should not be a problem if you restrict your workouts to those described in this book, and if you vary your workout regime as recommended.

Maintenance

If you have completed the intermediate IBC program described above and have decided that remaining at your current level satisfies your exercise goals, you have reached the fifth stage of exercise (chapter 8), maintenance. Your purpose now is to retain the gains you have already realized, without trying to progress to a higher intensity or workload. Maintenance at the intermediate level follows the same rules as the beginning level (chapter 4)—cross-training and periodization, but at a higher overall workload and intensity.

Graduation

You have come a long way. Your body weight is under control, you are harvesting all the health and wellness benefits of exercise, and you may even be approaching your perfect body. Where to now? That depends on you. Do you want to get as strong and fit as your genetics will allow? Do you want to explore your personal limits? Are you attracted to peak performance? Are you an athlete seeking to transition to a higher level? Are you a coach with the ambition and capacity to win a championship? If you answer affirmatively to any of these questions, you are a candidate for the advanced IBC program, to which we now turn.

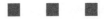

Appendix to Chapter 5

Health Screening and Cardiovascular Risk Stratification

Determining your cardiovascular risk level requires information about several car-diovascular risk factors, including your blood pressure, blood cholesterol, and fast-ing blood glucose. Obtain these data with the help of your doctor so you have all the information you need to complete the Cardiovascular Risk Factor Questionnaire on page 115. Your risk also depends on your body weight, measured by your Body Mass Index or BMI. Determine your BMI using your weight and height online using the Body Mass Index Calculator at www.MiracleWorkout.com, or calculate it your-self with the four-step procedure below.

After you have obtained your blood pressure, cholesterol levels, fasting blood glucose, and BMI, you are ready to answer the eight questions on the Cardiovascu-lar Risk Factor Questionnaire. Use the scoring directions following each question to enter the corresponding score onto the Cardiovascular Risk Factor Scorecard. You can also fill out the Cardiovascular Risk Factor Questionnaire online at www.MiracleWorkout.com, where your Risk Factor Score is computed automatically.

Calculating Your Body Mass Index

How do you know if you are underweight, overweight, or obese, and how much addi-tional cardiovascular risk does that entail? Find out by calculating your Body Mass Index (BMI) using the following four-step procedure (or using the automatic BMI calculator online), and then look up your associated risk factor in table 5.3.

First. Divide your weight in pounds by 2.2 to get your weight in kilograms.
Second. Multiply your height in inches by 0.0254 to get your height in meters.
Third. Square your height in meters (multiply it by itself).
Fourth. Divide your weight in kilograms (first step above) by your height in meters squared (third step above) to get your Body Mass Index in kilo-grams/meters squared.

Sample BMI Calculation

Suppose you weigh 142 pounds and are 5 feet 6 inches (66 inches) tall.

1. 142 pounds divided by 2.2 kilograms/pounds = 64.55 kilograms
2. 66 inches times 0.0254 meters/inches = 1.676 meters
3. 1.676 meters times 1.676 meters = 2.81 meters squared
4. 64.55 kilograms divided by 2.81 meters squared = 22.97 kilograms/meters squared

Your Body Mass Index is 22.97 kilograms/meters squared. That places you in the mid-range of "normal" in weight.

Body Mass Indexes, Weight Categories, and Disease Risk

Use table 5.3 to determine the weight category implied by your BMI and, with your waist measurement, to interpret your cardiovascular risk relative to "normal." The risk associated with body weight is dependent in part on waist girth because more abdominal fat is an *independent* risk indicator signifying a greater than normal chance of developing cardiovascular problems.

You are now ready to determine your cardiovascular risk level (see also table 5.4). Start by answering the following questionnaire, and then enter the score to each question into the scorecard that follows.

TABLE 5.3
CARDIOVASCULAR DISEASE RISK

(higher numbers signify progressively greater risk compared to "normal")

		Waist Measurement	
BMI (kilograms/ meters squared)	Weight Category	Men < 102 cm (40 inches) Women< 88 cm (35 inches)	Men > 102 cm (40 inches) Women> 88 cm (35 inches)
<18.5	Underweight	—	—
18.5–24.9	Normal	—	—
25.0–29.9	Overweight	1	2
30.0–34.9	Obese	2	3
35.0–39.9	More obese	3	3
>40.0	Extremely obese	4	4

Adapted from S. Going and R. Davis, "Body composition." From American College of Sports Medicine, *ACSM's Resource Manual for Guidelines for Exercise Testing and Prescription,* fourth edition (Baltimore, MD: American College of Sports Medicine, 2001), table 45.1, p. 393. Source: National Heart, Lung, and Blood Institute, National Institutes of Health, and U.S. Department of Health and Human Services.

CARDIOVASCULAR RISK FACTOR QUESTIONNAIRE

Answer the following questions about the indicated cardiovascular risk factor and score each answer following the directions at the end of each question. Sum your total risk factors on the scorecard (see next page), and read on for interpretation of your score.

YES NO

☐ ☐ **1. Family History.** Has any *male* first-degree relative (i. e., father, brother, son) experienced a myocardial infarction (heart attack), coronary revascularization (bypass surgery), or sudden death before the age of 55; *or* has any *female* first-degree relative (i.e., mother, sister, daughter) experienced a heart attack, bypass surgery, or sudden death before the age of 65? (Answer yes if *either* is true, no if *neither* is true.) *Scorecard directions:* if yes, enter +1; if no, enter 0.

☐ ☐ **2. Cigarette Smoking.** Are you currently a cigarette smoker or have you been a cigarette smoker during the last six months? *Scorecard directions:* if yes enter, +1; if no, enter 0.

☐ ☐ **3. High Blood Pressure.** Is your systolic blood pressure equal to or greater than 140 mm Hg (confirmed on at least two occasions), *or* is your diastolic blood pressure equal to or greater than 90 mm Hg (confirmed on at least two occasions), *or* are you currently taking prescribed medication for high blood pressure? (Answer yes if *any* are true, no if *none* is true.) *Scorecard directions:* if yes, enter +1; if no, enter 0.

☐ ☐ **4. High Blood Cholesterol.** Is your *total* serum cholesterol greater than 200 mg/dL *or* is your *low-density* lipoprotein cholesterol greater than 130 mg/dL, *or* is your *high-density* lipoprotein cholesterol less than 35 mg/dL, *or* are you taking prescribed medication to lower your blood cholesterol? (Answer yes if *any* are true, no if *none* is true.) *Scorecard directions:* if yes, enter +1; if no, enter 0.

☐ ☐ **5. Impaired Fasting Blood Glucose.** Is your fasting blood glucose equal to or greater than 110 mg/dL (confirmed on at least two occasions)? *Scorecard directions:* if yes, enter +1; if no, enter 0.

☐ ☐ **6. Obesity.** Is your Body Mass Index equal to or greater than 30 kg/m^2, *or* is your waist measurement greater than 100 cm (39½ inches)? (Answer yes if *either* is true, no if *neither* is true.) *Scorecard directions:* if yes, enter +1; if no, enter 0.

☐ ☐ **7. Sedentary Lifestyle.** Do you participate in a regular exercise program *or* get at least 30 minutes of moderate exercise accumulated over the whole day, at least three days a week? *Scorecard directions:* if yes, enter 0; if no, enter +1.

☐ ☐ **8. Blood Cholesterol NEGATIVE Risk Factor.** Is your *high-density* lipoprotein (HDL) cholesterol greater than 60 mg/dL? *Scorecard directions:* if yes, enter *negative* 1: if no, enter 0.

Adapted from the Guidelines of the American College of Sports Medicine, *ACSM's Guidelines for Exercise Testing and Prescription,* sixth edition (Philadelphia: Lippincott Williams & Wilkins, 2000), table 2.1, p. 24. Copyright © 2000 by American College of Sports Medicine. Reproduced by permission of Lippincott Williams & Wilkins. Original source: Expert Panel on Detection, Evaluation, and Treatment of High Blood Cholesterol in Adults. Summary of the second report of the National Cholesterol Foundation Program (NCEP) expert panel on detection, evaluation, and treatment of high blood pressure in adults (Adult Treatment Panel II). *Journal of American Medical Association* 269 (1993), pp. 3015–3023. Adapted with permission.

CARDIOVASCULAR RISK FACTOR QUESTIONNAIRE SCORECARD

Enter +1 for a yes answer, or 0 for a no answer, to the first seven questions on the Cardiovascular Risk Factor Questionnaire. For the eighth question on the questionnaire, enter −1 for a yes answer, or 0 for a no answer.

Question 1: Family History   _____

Question 2: Cigarette Smoking   _____

Question 3: High Blood Pressure   _____

Question 4: High Blood Cholesterol   _____

Question 5: Impaired Fasting Blood Glucose   _____

Question 6: Obesity   _____

Question 7: Sedentary Lifestyle   _____

SUBTOTAL: _____

Question 8: Blood Cholesterol NEGATIVE Risk Factor   _____

TOTAL (including question 8):   _____

Note: Your TOTAL should be between −1 and +7. If not, recalculate your score.

You are in the *low risk category* (table 5.4) if and only if you meet all of the following three criteria:

1. You are *asymptomatic* (that is, if you answered no to all questions on the Symptoms Questionnaire in the appendix to chapter 4).
2. You are a man under 45 or a woman under 55.
3. Your Cardiovascular Risk Factor Questionnaire Scorecard score is no greater than one.

You are in the *moderate risk category* (table 5.4) if you are asymptomatic and meet *either* of the following criteria:

1. You are a man 45 years of age or older or a woman 55 years of age or older.
2. Your Cardiovascular Risk Factor Questionnaire Scorecard score is 2 or greater.

You are automatically assigned to the *high risk category* (table 5.4) if you are symptomatic, that is, if you answered yes to any question on the Symptoms Questionnaire in appendix to chapter 4, even though many yes answers have a benign explanation. If you did answer yes to any question on the Symptoms Questionnaire, clarify the issue with your doctor before you exercise.

Instructions for Use of Intermediate Miracle Workout Logs

There are two different workout logs in the appendix to chapter 5, prescribed and generic. The prescribed intermediate workout log is based on the nine resistance exercises shown in figure 5.3, while the generic intermediate workout log is based on whatever eight resistance exercises you choose, plus the essential core (abdominal) exercises. The instructions for using the intermediate logs are the same for both workouts, and similar to those for the beginning IBC workout described in the appendix to chapter 4. There are, however, some additions and options built into the intermediate logs, including spaces for recording cardiovascular data, and the option of using an advanced heart monitor to record your overall workout parameters during resistance training.

Start by getting familiar with the general form of the workout log you choose. Just as in the beginning logs, there are spaces at the top for personal information, followed now, however, by four boxes. Each log again has three separate columns for recording three workouts, distinguished by block shading. The first box at the top is for date and day; the second for recording your cardiovascular conditioning data. The third box is for cardiolift data, while the fourth is for recording overall workout parameters. Scan the headings of columns and rows in preparation for the instructions that follow. If you choose your own resistance exercise (generic log), include the abdominal core exercises as the last exercise you do (exercise 9).

Start by entering your name at the top if you wish, followed by the upper limit of your heart rate window for active rest, your lower vigorous heart rate training window limit, your upper limit, and your target (middle) vigorous value. Calculate these values as percentages of your maximum heart rate (HR_{MAX}, estimated by the formula 220 minus your age in years), and use the percentages indicated in table 4.1 to find your values. Round all of your values to the nearest five to make them easier to remember, and check them against the decadal ranges in table 5.1 to con-

TABLE 5.4
DEFINITION OF CARDIOVASCULAR RISK CATEGORIES

Low Risk	Moderate Risk	High Risk
Asymptomatic men under 45 and asymptomatic women under 55 (all no answers on the Symptoms Questionnaire), with a cardiovascular risk score (from the scorecard) no greater than 1. If you are in this group, you can do moderate or vigorous exercise without a medical examination or exercise test.	Asymptomatic men 45 years of age or older, and asymptomatic women 55 years of age or older (all no answers on the Symptoms Questionnaire), or anyone of any age with a cardiovascular risk score (from the Scorecard) of 2 or greater. If you are in this group, you can do *moderate* exercise without a medical examination or exercise test, but clarify your medical status with your physician before *vigorous* exercise.	Individuals who are symptomatic (any yes answer on the Symptoms Questionnaire) or who have a known cardiovascular, pulmonary, or metabolic disease, or belong to a special clinical population as defined in chapter 9. If you are in this group, clarify your medical status with your physician before you exercise.

Adapted from the Guidelines of the American College of Sports Medicine, *ACSM's Guidelines for Exercise Testing and Prescription,* sixth edition (Philadelphia: Lippincott Williams & Wilkins, 2000), box 2.2, p. 26. Copyright © 2000 by American College of Sports Medicine. Reproduced by permission of Lippincott Williams & Wilkins.

firm your calculations. For the intermediate (but not beginning) IBC workout you can also use the Heart Rate Reserve method to calculate your heart rate training window (chapter 6).

As you begin each workout, record the workout number, date, and day of the week in the top box. Start your heart monitor and do a 10-minute warm-up. Then record from your heart monitor the parameters of your warm-up under CARDIOVAS-CULAR CONDITIONING. Enter these data for your cardiovascular warm-up in the spaces provided, as follows. Under TIME, record the duration of your warm-up (10 minutes is prescribed, though you can opt to do more if you can do so comfortably); under PROGRAM, record the specific program indicated by your cardiovascular machine, if any. Under LEVEL, record the level of intensity of your cardiovascular workout, as indicated by the machine you use. For the treadmill, use running velocity as your level. Under KCALS/AV. HR, record the Kcals burned and your average heart rate during your warm-up, as recorded with your heart monitor. You will see your average heart rate adapt (decline) despite maintained or increased exercise intensity (level) during cardiovascular exercise, which is a great way to watch your heart grow stronger. If you are using nonmotorized cardio options, record only your time and Kilocalories/Average Heart Rate.

Then move to the resistance phase of your workout, the cardiolift, and record values in the next box labeled FREE WEIGHTS AND EXERCISE MACHINES. The instructions for using this part of the intermediate workout logs are identical to those for the beginning IBC workout as detailed in the appendix to chapter 4, with the exception that you will perform two sets of each exercise rather than one. The column labeled SETS provides you a place to make a check after you complete each set. Remembering how many sets you have done becomes more of an issue in the advanced IBC workout, where you do three or four sets of each resistance exercise.

Load and record the weight you will use for the leg press in your first workout (prescribed workout) or whatever exercise you chose to do first (generic workout). The empty sled (leg press machine) or bars (free weights) have a weight that should be included in the weight you record. Reset and start your heart monitor, and then do your first cardio-acceleration to elevate your heart rate into your vigorous heart rate training window. Then do 8–12 repetitions of the leg press (prescribed workout) or your first exercise (generic workout), recording the number of repetitions in the column labeled REPS. In the columns labeled PAIN and EXERT, record whether any pain you felt during the leg press was greater than *weak* (yes or no), and whether the exertion was greater than *strong* (yes or no). If both answers were no, increase the weight by 10 pounds for your next workout, or instead increase the repetitions by one or two. When you advance to 12 repetitions and are ready to progress, lower the repetitions back to 8 and increase the weight

Intermediate Miracle Workout Log, Cardiolift Phase, Prescribed

Name _____

CARDIOVASCULAR PARAMETERS AND HEART RATE TRAINING WINDOW

Active Rest _____ **BPM**
(55 percent HR_{MAX})

Lower _____ **BPM**
(70 percent HR_{MAX})

Upper _____ **BPM**
(89 percent HR_{MAX})

Target _____ **BPM**
(80 percent HR_{MAX})

WORKOUT# _____		WORKOUT# _____		WORKOUT# _____	
Date (m/d/y)	Day of Week	Date (m/d/y)	Day of Week	Date (m/d/y)	Day of Week

CARDIOVASCULAR CONDITIONING

Cardiovascular (Check)	Time (min)	Program	Level	KCals/ Av HR	Time (min)	Program	Level	KCals/ Av HR	Time (min)	Program	Level	KCals/ Av HR
Stair Stepper ☐												
Treadmill ☐												
Cycle ☐												
Other ☐												

FREE WEIGHTS AND EXERCISE MACHINES

Exercise	wt, lbs	reps 8–12	sets (2)	Pain > Weak (Y/N)	Exert > Strong (Y/N)	wt, lbs	reps 8–12	sets (2)	Pain > Weak (Y/N)	Exert > Strong (Y/N)	wt, lbs	reps 8–12	sets (2)	Pain > weak (Y/N)	Exert > strong (Y/N)
1. Leg Press															
2. Leg Extension															
3. Leg Flexion															
4. Lat Pull-Downs															
5. Bench Press															

Exercise	wt, lbs	reps 8–12	sets (2)	Pain > Weak (Y/N)	Exert > Strong (Y/N)	wt, lbs	reps 8–12	sets (2)	Pain > Weak (Y/N)	Exert > Strong (Y/N)	wt, lbs	reps 8–12	sets (2)	Pain > weak (Y/N)	Exert > strong (Y/N)
6. Overhead Press															
7. Arm Curls															
8. Triceps Extension															
9. Core (Abs)															

OVERALL WORKOUT PARAMETERS

WinTim/Av. HR/Kcal	/ /	/ /	/ /
Weight Before/After	/	/	/
Water Used (liters)			
Pa > We/ Exert > St?	/	/	/
Observations and Comments			

Do not use this Workout Log without following the information and safety guidelines contained in the book *The Miracle Workout*. The Miracle Workout, and its agents, assume no liability for persons who use this Workout Log or change their exercise or physical activity. Copyright © 2002 by W. Jackson Davis. This Workout Log may be reproduced without change for personal use only.

Intermediate Miracle Workout Log, Cardiolift Phase, Generic

Name _____

CARDIOVASCULAR PARAMETERS AND HEART RATE TRAINING WINDOW

Active Rest _____ BPM
(55 percent HR$_{MAX}$)

Lower _____ BPM
(70 percent HR$_{MAX}$)

Upper _____ BPM
(89 percent HR$_{MAX}$)

Target _____ BPM
(80 percent HR$_{MAX}$)

WORKOUT# _____		WORKOUT# _____		WORKOUT# _____	
Date (m/d/y)	Day of Week	Date (m/d/y)	Day of Week	Date (m/d/y)	Day of Week

CARDIOVASCULAR CONDITIONING

Cardiovascular (Check)	Time (min)	Program	Level	KCals/ Av HR	Time (min)	Program	Level	KCals/ Av HR	Time (min)	Program	Level	KCals/ Av HR
Stair Stepper ☐												
Treadmill ☐												
Cycle ☐												
Other ☐												

FREE WEIGHTS AND EXERCISE MACHINES

Exercise (Write In)	wt, lbs	reps 8–12	sets (2)	Pain > Weak (Y/N)	Exert > Strong (Y/N)	wt, lbs	reps 8–12	sets (2)	Pain > Weak (Y/N)	Exert > Strong (Y/N)	wt, lbs	reps 8–12	sets (2)	Pain > weak (Y/N)	Exert > strong (Y/N)
1.															
2.															
3.															
4.															
5.															

Exercise	wt, lbs	reps 8–12	sets (2)	Pain > Weak (Y/N)	Exert > Strong (Y/N)	wt, lbs	reps 8–12	sets (2)	Pain > Weak (Y/N)	Exert > Strong (Y/N)	wt, lbs	reps 8–12	sets (2)	Pain > weak (Y/N)	Exert > strong (Y/N)
6.															
7.															
8.															
9.															

OVERALL WORKOUT PARAMETERS

WinTim/Av. HR/Kcal	/	/	/	/	/	/
Weight Before/After	/		/		/	
Water Used (liters)						
Pa > We/ Exert > St?	/		/		/	
Observations and Comments						

Do not use this Workout Log without following the information and safety guidelines contained in the book *The Miracle Workout*. The Miracle Workout, and its agents, assume no liability for persons who use this Workout Log or change their exercise or physical activity. Copyright © 2002 by W. Jackson Davis. This Workout Log may be reproduced without change for personal use only.

by 10 pounds for big muscles or 5 pounds for small muscles. Record the new values of repetitions and weights in the space provided for the next workout before you move to the next exercise in your current workout. If the new value of repetitions or weights is an advance, circle it. That rewards your advance, and enables you to see at a glance at your workout logs how you are progressing over time.

If you answered yes to the question about perceived pain, record the same weight and repetitions for your next workout, and seek professional assistance to understand it before you continue or work out again. If you answered yes to the question about perceived exertion, record the same weight and repetitions for your next workout. You have just implemented the IBC method of progression, which will keep you advancing in comfort as fast as your genetics will allow and with minimum risk of injury.

Move to the next exercise, and follow the same pattern as for the leg press. Continue performing two sets of each exercise to the end of your workout, in each case recording the values of weight and repetitions you will use in your next workout based on your RPP and RPE. When you advance in exercises involving small-muscle groups (generally upper body exercises), increment your weight by 5 rather than 10 pounds. You can record either the weight (in pounds) or the number of plates you lift.

When you are finished with the resistance exercises, immediately stop your heart monitor and record the values from your heart monitor in the box labeled OVERALL WORKOUT PARAMETERS, which differs from the beginning logs. The first row, WINTIM/AV. HR/KCAL, refers to data recorded by your heart monitor. WINTIM (window time) is your total time in your cardiovascular heart rate training window during the cardiolift workout you just completed, which is recorded on advanced heart monitors such as the Polar A5. AV HR is your average heart rate during the cardiolift phase, while KCAL is the total Kilocalories burned during the cardiolift phase. Record these three values respectively from your heart monitor in the three sections of each cell demarcated by backslashes, as an indication of your workout intensity. Restart your heart monitor and do your ROM cooldown.

The WEIGHT BEFORE/AFTER row provides a place to record your body weight before and after you work out. If your weight is unchanged, you drank enough water. Record also the amount you drank in the next row (WATER USED [LITERS]), which will help you dial in the appropriate amount to drink.

The next row is labeled PA > WE, EXERT > ST? That's shorthand for is "Pain greater than *weak,* exertion greater than *strong*?" and pertains to the cumulative feeling you have at the end of your cardiolift workout. Enter yes or no for pain before the backslash, and for exertion after the backslash.

Then implement gating, by accepting or rejecting the advances you made in individual resistance exercises based on these answers. If your overall pain was greater than *weak,* stay at the same level next time in all individual exercises, and find out the cause of the pain with professional help as required. If your overall exertion was greater than *strong,* likewise remain at the same level in each individual exercise for your next workout. If you answered no to both these pain and exertion questions, accept all the advances you made in individual exercises for your next workout.

The OBSERVATIONS AND COMMENTS row is for recording any general impressions of your physical or emotional state following your workout. In addition, use this space to footnote the details of any pain that you experienced in any individual resistance exercise. That way you will have a record of how any particular pain behaved over time, which can help you understand and deal with persistent or repetitive pain.

■   ■   ■

6

Your Advanced Miracle Workout

The advanced IBC program confers all the benefits of the beginning and intermediate levels, including health, wellness, and top physical fitness. In addition, the
advanced workout adds a new dimension: peak performance. Athletes, this is your
conditioning program, both during your sport and in the off season. The workout
described in this chapter helped propel the University of California at Santa Cruz
(UCSC) men's soccer team to the national championships two years running, and
is now the foundation for training in the UCSC Athletic Department. The advanced
IBC program is not just for athletes, however—it is for anyone at any age with the
curiosity, courage, and will to seek and push their limits.

Peak performance is an important tool for many in quest of excellence, in or
out of the gym. The advanced IBC program is for you at any age if you are already
in very good physical condition and you wonder how far you can go. If you are
already a dedicated exerciser frustrated by stagnation and plateaus, or simply by
the boredom of your current exercise program (see the following sidebar), the
advanced workout will help you break the pattern. If you are a senior citizen,
peak performance may mean attaining the cardiovascular conditioning, strength,
and endurance of a younger person, or doing activities you had long since given
up. This workout is for you if you are motivated, disciplined, and excited to
explore the boundaries of your being. The challenge is high, and the rewards
enormous.

Myth Buster 6: Exercise Is Bo-o-o-oring

THE MYTH: Exercise is a recipe for boredom.

If you review the testimonials in chapter 3 to see how users feel about IBC, the first thing that stands out is how many people say they like it because it is so engaging. Time flies during an IBC workout, which is one reason most people prefer IBC to any other conventional exercise approach we've tried.

Several features of IBC combat boredom, starting with cardio-driving. You'll never just sit around waiting to get ready for exercise in IBC—instead, and as you've perhaps experienced by now, you are always on the move from cardio to resistance to Range of Motion exercise and back again. It is a very proactive workout.

Then there is the constant exercise of the mind–body connection. An IBC workout is an exercise in body awareness, that alone keeps you from getting bored. You'll monitor constantly your exertion level, any pain you feel, your heart rate, the weights and repetitions you do—there is simply no time for boredom.

Then there are motivational tools such as peak performance goals for additional interest (chapter 8), cross-training for variation, periodization over the year, the outdoor workouts for sheer pleasure, and—powering it all—the seductive runner's high . . .

Conventional exercise can be boring, even excruciatingly dull. In contrast, IBC engages the full human capacities like few forms of exercise—mind, heart, and body all work together, seamlessly, with the consequence that time flies so fast, and the workout is so much fun, that boredom is never an issue.

THE REALITY: IBC is the most engaging exercise program you'll ever do. You won't have time to get bored.

The IBC Myth Buster

MYTH: Exercise is boring.

FACT: For most people, IBC is the most enjoyable and exciting workout ever developed.

Safety at the Edge

You can tell you are ready for the advanced IBC workout if you can exercise comfortably at the end point of the intermediate workout—that is, you can do vigorous integrated exercise for 50 minutes in comfort. If that description does not fit your current physical condition, return to chapter 5 and follow the intermediate IBC program until you reach this relatively high level of cardiovascular conditioning. The advanced IBC program entails intense exercise for a minimum of 90 minutes, and for as long as two or more continuous hours. You will not only sustain a high heart rate, but also lift heavy weights repeatedly. Total workload in a single two-hour advanced workout can reach 40 tons or more. Physical activity at this level can increase eightfold the volume of blood your heart pumps and cause transient elevations of blood pressure up to two or more times normal resting levels.

The recommended safety preparations of the American College of Sports Medicine (ACSM) for vigorous exercise include health screening and cardiovascular risk stratification (chapter 5). If this process places you in the moderate- or high-risk category, the ACSM recommends a current medical examination and physician-supervised maximal exercise test before you begin vigorous exercise. Both may be advisable anyway, regardless of your cardiovascular risk level, and particularly if you are older (men 45 or older, women 55).

Two additional safety tools can help minimize pain and maximize gain from your advanced IBC program. The first is a detailed health and medical history. According to Dr. Michael C. Koester, a leading expert in pediatric sports, "More than 90 percent of problems that limit [athletic] participation [in youth] can be determined through a good history."[1] Past injuries and surgeries are important because they create a physiological weak point that is vulnerable to repeat injury. Consequently, they are among your most important leading indicators of unnecessary and avoidable pain and injury—and interruption of your training program.

You can record your health and medical history using the Health, Medical History, and Physical Activity Form posted at www.MiracleWorkout.com (click on "Safety/Advanced"). The most common issues are bone and joint problems, usually from previous surgeries or injuries, and asthma.* Athletes that we train fill this form out for the record, and then update it as appropriate.†

We record the relevant health or medical history issue on 3-by-5-inch cards for reference during training, creating flags to follow every issue. You can use a similar procedure during your workouts as follows:

---

* Past bone and joint injuries are particularly vulnerable to reinjury. If you have asthma, get your doctor's advice about prolonged vigorous exercise, and always carry an inhaler during workouts.

† If you are an exercise professional or trainer, or if you are an agent of an institution such as a health club, review provisions of the Health Insurance Portability and Accountability Act (HIPAA) of 2002 before you collect, use, or hold personal medical information of other people. Visit the Symantec website at www. symantec.com, and click on Synaptic Enterprise Industry Web Sites/Solutions for Related Security tools.

- Clarify every significant health or medical history issue with your doctor or trainer, and record each on a 3-by-5-inch card.
- Tape each card to your workout clipboard beneath your workout logs to flag the issue, and review each flag at the start of every workout to raise your consciousness about the issue.
- Read and monitor every flag as part of every workout, and before every exercise pertinent to the flag.
- Record any change in every flagged condition on the card and date it so you can follow it over time. Seek professional or medical advice for any condition that causes you any pain or changes over time.

Your second and related tool for minimizing the risk of injury is an effective strategy for managing pain. Unless you are a young nonathlete, some degree of pain at advanced exercise levels may be inevitable. If you are a competitive athlete, pain comes with the territory. If you are a senior and have led an active life, you've no doubt earned those aches and pains. Dr. Abraham Verghese writes that pain from exercise has become a kind of status symbol of active elders, "the emblem of the new virtue"[2] of exercise. True, but pain is also a warning, which if unheeded can interrupt or end your exercise program.

Managing pain effectively requires navigating between the extremes of unacceptable pain that you treat immediately, and unavoidable pain that you may have to grin and bear to exercise at all. Unacceptable pain includes the exercise stop signs—chest, head, or abdominal pain, as well as dizziness (chapter 4), and overuse symptoms and injuries (chapter 5). Unavoidable pain includes the everyday aches and pains that you can work through, shortness of breath, and minor sports injuries. Use these four criteria to help tell the difference and always seek professional advice:

1. Intensity.
   Determine the cause of any pain that feels greater than *weak,* as part of the IBC method of progression. Any pain intense enough to interfere with sleep merits attention. Only when you understand a pain can you make an intelligent decision about whether to work through it. Past injuries, as well as the aging process, leave some exercisers little choice but to work through some pain that may register as greater than *weak.* Make any such choice, however, only with the advice of your doctor or trainer.
2. Persistence.
   Any pain that does not disappear after one or two days, including weak pain, requires action. It could signify an overuse injury. If the pain worsens, it

deserves immediate evaluation and perhaps even a different approach to exercise. Certain kinds of pain—particularly knee, pelvic, and lower back—can start out barely perceptible and then grow over a period of 24–48 hours. With experience, you learn to recognize these sleepers. In the meantime, be wary of even apparently minor twinges in these vulnerable areas, particularly if they occur during resistance exercise at higher overload weights.

3. **Distribution.**

   Pain in just one spot or on one side (unilateral) merits further attention because it may signify injury. Some forms of bilateral pain—those that are weak and short lived—are less problematic, including mild, bilateral muscle soreness. After your first couple of IBC workouts, however, muscle soreness should never be an issue.

4. **Type.**

   Joint pain always deserves a closer look. Joints are primary weak links, particularly as we age, and are easy to injure and slow to heal. Any persistent pain or swelling at any joint requires professional evaluation, whether localized (unilateral) or more general (bilateral). Joint swelling can be symptomatic of rheumatoid arthritis, which requires special care and medical evaluation during exercise. Head, chest, or abdominal pain are always warnings to stop exercise immediately and get advice. A side stitch or muscle "burn" during repetitions is not generally a problem.

Here is a simple three-step strategy that incorporates these criteria to keep your IBC program moving without interruption and to minimize the risk of injury:

1. Evaluate the *intensity* of any pain using the RPP scale. Any pain greater than *weak* requires understanding before you continue.
2. Determine the *distribution* of any pain. In addition to the stop signs, any pain that is unilateral, localized, or in joints requires a closer look.
3. Assess the *persistence* of pain, and seek professional advice for any pain that does not disappear in a day or two or that keeps you awake.

The Blueprint for Your Advanced IBC Program

The advanced IBC program follows the three-step pattern that is by now familiar (figure 6.1). We'll continue to describe the gym workout for consistency. The advanced workout adds two resistance exercises to the intermediate workout, however, and employs three sets rather than two of each resistance exercise during the cardiolift. The advanced workout also adds three ROM exercises. When you can do vigorous

FIGURE 6.1
THE THREE-STEP ADVANCED IBC PROGRAM MADE SIMPLE

1. **Prerequisites.** Excellent physical condition, low cardiovascular risk category (see appendix, or www.MiracleWorkout.com, click on "Safety" and then "Advanced"), or medical clearance. Recommended: health and medical history (see text), current medical exam, doctor-supervised maximal exercise test.
2. **Intensity.** Prolonged vigorous exercise.
3. **Description.** Three steps: two preparatory and one integrated.

Step 1: Cardio (preparatory)

1. **Goal.** 60 minutes of vigorous cardio exercise in complete comfort.
2. **Method.** Self-paced, progressive aerobic (cardio) exercise.
3. **Time.** 60 minutes per workout, three workouts per week, for two to four weeks.

Step 2: Cardiorom (preparatory, partially integrated)

1. **Goal.** Integration of ROM with prolonged vigorous cardio exercise.
2. **Method.** Alternate vigorous cardio and ROM exercise.
3. **Time.** 60 minutes per workout, three workouts per week, for two to four weeks.

Step 3: Cardiolift (fully integrated)

1. **Goal.** Integration of weightlifting with prolonged vigorous cardio exercise followed by ROM cooldown.
2. **Method.** Alternate cardio and weightlifting exercise with a terminal ROM cooldown.
3. **Time.** 90 minutes or more per workout, two to three workouts per week, indefinite to cross-training, periodization, or taper for sports season.

cardio exercise comfortably for 60 continuous minutes, integrate flexibility and resistance exercises into your cardio routine in two stages, cardiorom and cardiolift. For a transitional workout, you can do the exercises in this chapter using two rather than three sets.

An Advanced Measure of Exercise Intensity

There are significant differences between the intermediate and advanced IBC programs. The first is the way you determine your heart rate training window. You still work at vigorous intensity, just as at the intermediate level, but you use a different method to calculate it, termed the Heart Rate Reserve (HRR) method or the Karvonen method after its founder. The HRR method is more accurate, particularly for advanced or older exercisers, but you can also use it to determine your heart rate training window at the intermediate level. Avoid using the HRR method at beginning levels, however, where the maximum heart rate method is more appropriate.

To apply the HRR method, measure your resting heart rate when you awaken in the morning before you get out of bed. Subtract your resting heart rate from your maximum heart rate (220 minus your age in years) to get your HRR. Multiply your HRR by 0.6 (table 6.1) and add back your resting heart rate to get the lower boundary of your vigorous heart rate training window. Multiply your HRR by 0.84 and add back your resting heart rate to get the upper limit of your training window. Round off each value to the nearest five to make your vigorous heart rate training window easier to remember. Here are the formulae:

TABLE 6.1
HEART RATE RANGES FOR EXERCISE OF DIFFERENT INTENSITIES BASED ON THE HEART RATE RESERVE METHOD

Exercise Intensity Level	Percent of Heart Rate Reserve
Very light	<20%
Light	20–39%
Moderate	40–59%
Hard (vigorous)	60–84%
Very hard (heavy)	≥85%
Maximal	100%

From American College of Sports Medicine, *ACSM's Guidelines for Exercise Testing and Prescription,* sixth edition (Philadelphia: Lippincott Williams & Wilkins, 2000), table 7-2, p. 150. Adapted originally from M. L. Pollock, G. A. Gaesser, J. D. Butcher, et al. "The Recommended Quantity and Quality of Exercise for Developing and Maintaining Cardiorespiratory and Muscular Fitness, and Flexibility in Healthy Adults." *Med Sci Sports Exerc* 30 (1998), pp. 975–991. Copyright © 2000 by American College of Sports Medicine. Reproduced by permission of Lippincott Williams & Wilkins.

$$\text{HRR Lower Boundary} = (\text{HR}_{\text{MAX}} - \text{HR}_{\text{REST}})\,(0.6) + \text{HR}_{\text{REST}}$$

$$\text{HRR Upper Boundary} = (\text{HR}_{\text{MAX}} - \text{HR}_{\text{REST}})\,(0.84) + \text{HR}_{\text{REST}}$$

Where HR_{MAX} = your maximum heart rate = 220 – your age in years and

HR_{REST} = your resting heart rate

Here's a sample calculation. Julie is 47 years of age, and an experienced and well-conditioned exerciser. Her resting heart rate on awakening is 60 Beats per Minute (BPM). Julie's Heart Rate Reserve is her estimated maximum heart rate (220 minus her age, or 173 BPM) minus her resting heart rate (60 BPM), or 113 BPM. The lower boundary of Julie's vigorous heart rate training window is:

$$(173 \text{ BPM} - 60 \text{ BPM})\,(0.6) + 60 \text{ BPM}$$

$$= (113 \times 0.6) + 60 = 127.8$$

$$= 130 \text{ (rounded to the nearest five)}$$

The upper boundary of her vigorous heart rate training window is:

$$(173 \text{ BPM} - 60 \text{ BPM})\,(0.84) + 60 \text{ BPM}$$

$$= (113 \times 0.84) + 60 = 154.9$$

$$= 155 \text{ (rounded to the nearest five)}$$

Julie's vigorous heart rate training window, determined by the HRR method, is therefore 130–155 BPM. Note that this range is slightly different from her vigorous heart rate training window calculated by the maximum heart rate method (120–155 BPM). Using the more physiologically realistic HRR method, she exercises in a higher heart rate training window, giving her a better workout that is more appropriate to her superior physical condition.

HRR calculations for vigorous exercise are shown in table 6.2 for 10-year age increments and for three different resting heart rates—50, 60, and 70 BPM. Lower heart rate is associated with better cardiorespiratory fitness. For men, 50, 60, and 70 BPM resting heart rates correspond approximately to excellent, good, and average physical condition. Women have slightly higher average heart rates than men, so resting heart rates of 50, 60, and 70 BPM in women correspond approximately to

TABLE 6.2
VIGOROUS EXERCISE HEART RATE WINDOWS FOR DIFFERENT AGES BASED ON THE HEART RATE RESERVE METHOD (60–84% HRR)

Age (years)	Maximum Heart Rate (220 – age)	Resting Heart Rate 50 BPM	Resting Heart Rate 60 BPM	Resting Heart Rate 70 BPM
10	210	145–185	150–185	155–190
20	200	140–175	145–180	150–180
30	190	135–170	140–170	140–170
40	180	130–160	130–160	135–160
50	170	120–150	125–150	130–155
60	160	115–140	120–145	125–145
70	150	110–135	115–135	120–135
80	140	105–125	110–125	110–130
90	130	100–115	100–120	105–120
100	120	90–110	95–110	100–110

Calculated values in ranges are rounded off to the nearest five. The ranges shown assume you are not taking any medications or substances that may influence your heart rate up or down, or otherwise interact adversely with vigorous exercise. If in doubt, consult your doctor.

superb, excellent, and good physical condition. After you calculate your vigorous heart rate training window using the HRR method, corroborate your values against those shown in table 6.2. The numbers shown there again assume that you are not taking any medication or substance that influences your heart rate, or otherwise interacts adversely with vigorous exercise. If you have doubts, get your doctor's advice.

A second, optional refinement in the way you calculate your heart rate training window in the advanced IBC program involves your maximum heart rate. For the beginning and intermediate levels, 220 minus your age is a satisfactory approximation. That formula works at the advanced level, too, but it can deviate from your true maximum heart rate by 10 BPM or more. Moreover, the 220 – age formula becomes progressively less accurate as you age or get into better physical condition, with the effect that you may be exercising progressively lower in your true heart rate training window. It's more accurate, but also riskier, to measure your maximum heart rate directly using the maximal exercise test.

Approach a maximal exercise test with caution even if you are in excellent aerobic condition. Make sure you fall into the low-risk cardiovascular category (chapter 5), and if you are a man older than 45, or a woman older than 55, consult your physician first. Avoid a maximal exercise test if you are pregnant or if you belong to any other special clinical population (chapter 9). For safety, we also recommend supervision by your physician or an exercise professional certified in CPR. On the other hand, the rewards of increased accuracy can be substantial.*

If you and your doctor decide a maximal exercise test is right for you, make sure you have had plenty of sleep, have eaten well, and have not exercised heavily for the past two days. Wear your normal workout clothing and your heart monitor. Warm up for 10 minutes, and then, over the next 10 minutes, increase your exercise intensity in 2-minute stages until you reach your maximum exercise level. That occurs when your heart rate no longer increases with further increments in exercise intensity, which typically occurs at an RPE between *very strong* and *extremely strong*. Compare the maximum heart rate you measure to the value you obtain from the 220 – age formula, and use whichever value is greater to calculate your heart rate training window. Recalculate your training window every several weeks during advanced training to ensure you continue to exercise in the window that confers maximum benefit.

Using the HRR method described above, calculate your heart rate training value for active rest (40 percent of your HRR, the lower boundary of your moderate exercise range), and your window for vigorous exercise (60–84 percent of HRR; table 6.1). Confirm that your values are in the right range from table 6.2.

---

* The 220 – age formula gives my maximum heart rate as 158 BPM, but my measured maximum heart rate is 185 BPM. My resting heart rate is 50 BPM, so when I use my maximum heart rate as estimated from the 220 – age formula to calculate my vigorous heart rate training window with the HRR method, it is 115–140 BPM. When I use my maximum heart rate of 185 measured from a maximal exercise test, however, the HRR method gives me a more accurate vigorous heart rate training window of 130–165 BPM. If I used the 220 – age estimate, therefore, I would be exercising well below my capacity, and impeding development correspondingly.

FIGURE 6.2
THE RATING OF PERCEIVED PAIN (RPP) MEASURING SCALE

Use this quantitative scale to evaluate any pain you feel during your IBC workout, following the instructions below.

Rating	Subjective Feeling
0	Nothing at all (no soreness/other pain)
0.3	
0.5	Extremely weak (just noticeable soreness/other pain)
0.7	
1	Very weak
1.5	
2	Weak (light intensity soreness/other pain)
2.5	
3	Moderate
4	
5	Strong (heavy intensity soreness/other pain)
6	
7	Very strong
8	
9	
10	Extremely strong (strongest-intensity soreness/other pain)
11	
•	Absolute maximum (highest-possible-intensity soreness/other pain)

Instructions for use: During the exercise . . . pay close attention to any pain you may feel anywhere in your body, including muscle soreness, joint, or trunk pain. Concentrate on the pain and estimate its intensity using the above scale. Try not to underestimate or overestimate your feeling of pain; be as accurate as you can.

From Gunnar Borg, *G. Borg's Perceived Exertion and Pain Scales* (Champaign, IL: Human Kinetics, 1998). Reproduced with author permission.

FIGURE 6.3
THE RATING OF PERCEIVED EXERTION MEASURING SCALE

Use this quantitative scale at the end of each resistance exercise and your whole workout to assess how much exertion they took to complete (see text).

Rating	Subjective Feeling
0	Nothing at all (no intensity)
0.3	
0.5	Extremely weak (just noticeable)
0.7	
1	Very weak
1.5	
2	Weak (light intensity)
2.5	
3	Moderate
4	
5	Strong (heavy intensity)
6	
7	Very strong
8	
9	
10	Extremely strong (strongest intensity)
11	
•	Absolute maximum (highest possible intensity)

Instructions for use: During the exercise . . . pay close attention to how hard you feel the exercise work rate is. This feeling should reflect your total amount of exertion and fatigue, combining all sensations and feelings of physical stress, effort, and fatigue. Don't concern yourself with any one factor such as leg pain, shortness of breath, or exercise intensity, but try to concentrate on your total, inner feeling of exertion. Try not to underestimate or overestimate your feeling of exertion; be as accurate as you can.

From Gunnar Borg, *G. Borg's Perceived Exertion and Pain Scales* (Champaign, IL: Human Kinetics, 1998). Reproduced with author permission.

The Advanced Method of Progression

Progression in the advanced cardio workout is based on your Rating of Perceived Pain (RPP) and Rating of Perceived Exertion (RPE), just as in the beginning and intermediate workouts. If you keep workout logs (appendix to this chapter), record your RPP and RPE as numerical values (figures 6.2 and 6.3). If your RPP is 2 (*weak*) or less (figure 6.2) and your RPE is 5 (*strong*) or less (figure 6.3), progress—add time to your next cardio workout, or add repetitions or weights to your next cardiolift. If your RPP was more than 2, however, make sure you understand the cause of the pain as soon as possible but certainly before your next workout, and then repeat the same workout next time. Likewise, if your RPE exceeded 5, repeat the same workout next time.

The Advanced Cardio Workout

As you start your advanced cardio workout, you'll find that your heart rate increases more slowly than when you were less fit. That's because your heart has greater pumping power, so it need not beat as fast. Use your heart monitor to watch your heart rate climb into your training range. If you experience any pain at all, evaluate it immediately using the quantitative RPP scale (figure 6.2), which puts numbers on the now familiar self-measurement categories. After 20 minutes of vigorous exercise in your first advanced cardio workout, cool down for the next few minutes. Gradually bring your heart rate down to the active rest level of 40 percent of your HRR—the lower boundary of moderate-intensity exercise. An ideal way to cool down is by stretching and bending without intermittent cardio acceleration. This cooldown is an integral part of every advanced workout, for the same reasons as in the beginning and intermediate workouts.

Follow the advanced method of progression described above, incrementing your aerobic time by 5 minutes each time your RPP is equal to 2 or less, and your RPE is equal to 5 or less. Keep progressing until you can do 60 continuous minutes of vigorous cardio exercise in full comfort. That may take from one to a few weeks, depending on your initial condition. When you can do vigorous aerobic exercise continuously for an hour without undue exertion (RPE$\leq$5) or pain (RPP$\leq$2), determined using the RPP and RPE scales shown in figures 6.2 and 6.3, you are ready to move the advanced cardiorom workout.

The Advanced Cardiorom Workout

The main difference from the intermediate cardiorom is that you have more time—up to 90 minutes. This enables you to include more ROM exercises. Figure 6.4

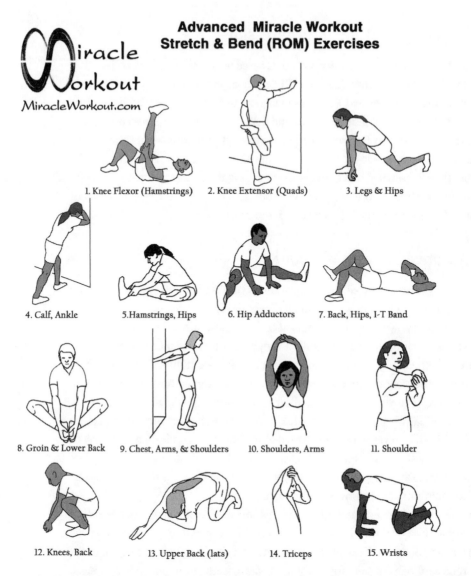

Advanced Miracle Workout
Stretch & Bend (ROM) Exercises

Miracle Workout
MiracleWorkout.com

1. Knee Flexor (Hamstrings) 2. Knee Extensor (Quads) 3. Legs & Hips

4. Calf, Ankle 5. Hamstrings, Hips 6. Hip Adductors 7. Back, Hips, I-T Band

8. Groin & Lower Back 9. Chest, Arms, & Shoulders 10. Shoulders, Arms 11. Shoulder

12. Knees, Back 13. Upper Back (lats) 14. Triceps 15. Wrists

Do not use this Worksheet without following the information and safety guidelines contained in the book *The Miracle Workout*. The Miracle Workout, and its agents, assume no liability for persons who use this Worksheet or change their exercise or physical activity. Copyright © 2004 by W. Jackson Davis. This Worksheet may be reproduced for personal use only.

FIGURE 6.4 **Advanced IBC Stretch and Bend (ROM) Exercises** This advanced sequence of Range of Motion exercises adds to the intermediate sequence shown in figure 5.2. Three new ROM exercises are added, for the groin and lower back (exercise 8), shoulders (exercise 11), and knees and back (exercise 12). You can add or substitute your own ROM exercises so long as your routine stays balanced across opposing muscle groups and across the whole body. Warm up before stretching and bending to minimize the risk of injury.

contains a basic set of ROM exercises suitable for advanced applications, including the same ROM exercises that you did at the intermediate level and three new stretching exercises. These 15 ROM exercises engage all primary, secondary, and tertiary body joints, ensuring a balanced workout. As an advanced exerciser, however, you can design your personal ROM routine. Create your own ROM program, or several that you can do in alternate workouts, from the vast range of ROM exercises available. If you are an athlete, consider a sequence tailored to your sport.

The beginning and intermediate cardiorom each started with a brief warm-up. You have more time now, and you're in better physical shape, so you're ready to take advantage of a new feature of the IBC workout. Extend your vigorous warm-up to a 20-minute vigorous heat-up, with these benefits:

- Blood circulation to your muscles increases dramatically, feeding and cleansing your muscles more effectively.
- The internal temperature of your muscles climbs 100-fold in comparison with a short warm-up,* loosening fascia, tendons, and ligaments, and accelerating all of the biochemical processes that underlie muscle contraction.
- The sweat response starts at about the 15-minute mark, accompanied by the runner's high that energizes the subsequent ROM or resistance exercises.
- The heat-up pre-fatigues your cardiovascular system, helping to keep your heart rate from recovering too fast during each subsequent set of ROM or resistance exercise.

Following your heat-up, progress through the cardiorom sequence as you did at the intermediate level. Keep your heart rate in your vigorous heart rate training window, based on the HRR method, by intermittent cardio-acceleration, and complete each ROM exercise while your heart rate remains in your training window. Hold each ROM position for 15–30 seconds, and continue until you have finished the 15 ROM exercises shown in figure 6.4, or whatever other ROM exercise sequence you select. You should finish your ROM routine in about 40 minutes, including the intermittent cardio-acceleration bouts. Taking into account the time for your heat-up, you'll have plenty of time left for your active cooldown, in which

---

* A conventional 5- or 10-minute vigorous warm-up raises temperature in the working muscle(s) by less than 0.1 degree Celsius, while a 30-minute heat-up increases the temperature of the same muscle by a remarkable 10 degrees C.

your heart rate settles down to the active rest level of 40 percent of your HRR over 5 or 10 minutes. You should be able to complete your advanced cardiorom in about an hour.*

Progress through the cardiorom workout by increasing the intensity of your initial heat-up and the intermittent cardio-acceleration bouts. You can also increase the hold time of each ROM exercise to 30 seconds or even longer, and repeat each ROM exercise up to a total of three or more stretches. Employ the strategies outlined in chapter 5 to counter rapid heart rate recovery—increase the duration and intensity of your heat-up and the intermittent cardio-accelerations. Your RPP and RPE (figures 6.2 and 6.3) again regulate your rate of progression, as at the intermediate level. When you can do a full advanced cardiorom session while sustaining your heart rate in your vigorous heart rate training window for a minimum of 60 minutes with an RPP no greater than 2 and an RPE no greater than 5, you're ready to move to the cardiolift phase.

The Advanced Cardiolift Workout

The first difference you will notice with the intermediate cardiolift is the longer workout time—90 minutes instead of 60—broken down into 20–60–10 minutes for the heat-up, cardiolift, and ROM cooldown, respectively. The advanced cardiolift is also more work, for three reasons.

1. You work at a higher level of intensity in your vigorous heart rate training window.
2. You add more resistance exercises.
3. You perform three sets of each weightlifting exercise rather than the two sets you did in the intermediate cardiolift.

The resistance exercises used in the advanced cardiolift need be no different from the ones you used in the intermediate workout. The greater time available for weightlifting—60 rather than 40 minutes—means you can add a couple of exercises, however, and remain within the time limit. Figure 6.5 shows a sequence of basic resistance exercises similar to the workout we used to train the championship men's soccer team at the University of California (chapter 3).

Figure 6.5 contains the resistance exercises you did in the intermediate IBC

---

* Twenty minutes for your heat-up, fifteen 1-minute intermittent cardio-driving bouts, fifteen ROM exercises at a minute each, 5 minutes of transaction time, and a 5-minute cooldown, for a total workout time of about one hour.

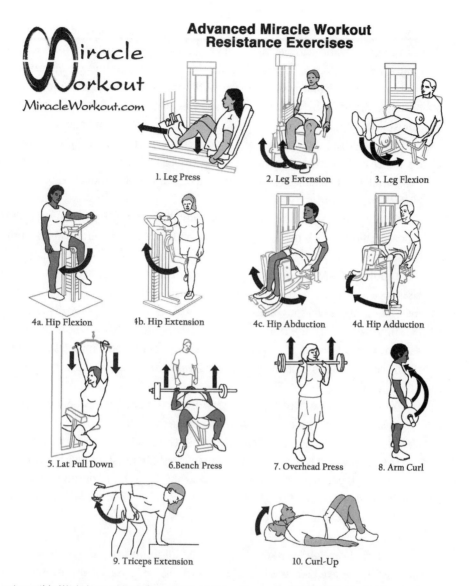

Advanced Miracle Workout Resistance Exercises

Miracle Workout
MiracleWorkout.com

1. Leg Press

2. Leg Extension

3. Leg Flexion

4a. Hip Flexion

4b. Hip Extension

4c. Hip Abduction

4d. Hip Adduction

5. Lat Pull Down

6. Bench Press

7. Overhead Press

8. Arm Curl

9. Triceps Extension

10. Curl-Up

Do not use this Worksheet without following the information and safety guidelines contained in the book *The Miracle Workout*. The Miracle Workout, and its agents, assume no liability for persons who use this Worksheet or change their exercise or physical activity. Copyright © 2004 by W. Jackson Davis. This Worksheet may be reproduced for personal use only.

FIGURE 6.5 **Advanced IBC Resistance Exercises** Here is an advanced sequence of resistance exercises that extends the intermediate sequence shown in figure 5.4. The advanced sequence adds exercises for the hips (figure 6.5, exercises 4a–4d). As before, arrows show the direction, range, and trajectory or arc of the concentric phase of each movement. See the safety tips for weightlifting exercises in chapter 4.

program, plus four new hip exercises (exercises 4a–4d). You can add these hip exercises to the advanced resistance sequence and keep within the 60-minute time limit if your gym has a hip machine like the one shown in figure 6.5, exercise 4a. Do hip abduction and adduction using this same machine, with no pause for cardio-acceleration between the four exercises. The hip muscles are large enough to sustain a robust heart rate, so as you move directly from one hip exercise to the next, your heart rate should remain in your training window. At three sets for each resistance exercise with brief cardio-accelerations between, you should just be able to finish the 10 resistance exercises (figure 6.5) in the 60 minutes available on the 20–60–10 timetable.

Create a more varied advanced workout by substituting more specialty or sport-specific exercises tailored to your own preferences and exercise goals. Some of the additional exercises illustrated in the last chapter (figure 5.4), for example, may meet your needs. At the advanced level, you are also ready to add extra core exercises such as the bench squat and dead lift, which work the spinal erectors. If it's too much for a single workout, consider split cardiolift sessions—lower body/core one day, upper body/core the next—or design entirely different workouts for different days. You may also want to add different exercises for the same muscles to stimulate them with a different neuromuscular coordination pattern and accelerate your development.

You have now selected and learned your sequence of 10 resistance exercises for the advanced cardiolift, and mastered the elements of form—support, movement, and breathing, including the double-breathing method (chapter 5), which you will need at the advanced level. You are ready to integrate resistance with cardiovascular exercise. If you record your workouts—which is useful at the advanced level—use the workout logs in the appendix to this chapter, which are also downloadable in 8½-by-11-inch format from www.MiracleWorkout.com (click on "Workout Logs").

Your first cardiolift workout begins with a 20-minute heat-up. Then set up your first resistance exercise, the leg press (figure 6.5, exercise 1). During setup, your heart rate will fall out of your vigorous training window, accelerated by your now higher level of physical conditioning. Do a quick cardio-acceleration to raise it back into your window. Introduce variation by switching among the cardio machines, and among motorized and nonmotorized options (chapter 4). Do your first resistance exercise, the leg press (exercise 1) while your heart rate is still elevated into your vigorous heart rate training window. Adjust your weights and repetitions according to your comfort level and exercise goals (table 5.2), but 8–12 repetitions is a good middle range. Following your first set of leg presses, do another cardio-acceleration and then a second set of the same leg press exercise. After another cardio-acceleration, do a third set of the same exercise using the same number of repetitions. Two sets of resistance exercises grow you faster and stronger than one, and three are better than two.

When you complete your third set of leg presses, dismantle your weights, wipe the chair dry, hydrate, and move to your second exercise station. Continue through the remaining resistance exercises, completing the entire sequence shown in figure 6.5 or your own customized routine. Remember to double the repetitions for core exercises (16–24 repetitions per set for three sets). After you know your weightlifting routine well, you should be able to finish the cardiolift workout in about 60 minutes.* You have 10 minutes left in your 90-minute workout to cool down, using the same ROM sequence you did in the cardiorom phase (30 seconds per stretch) with no interpolated cardio exercise. During your ROM cooldown, decrease your heart rate steadily to about 40 percent of your HRR, the lower boundary of your moderate exercise activity level. That will complete the cardiolift phase of your intermediate IBC workout in the 90-minute target time.[†]

Gating Your Advances

As soon as you finish your cooldown, evaluate your whole-workout RPP and RPE, and record the numeric values. Use these elements of biofeedback to gate the individual advances in weight or repetition that you recorded in resistance exercises, as described for the intermediate workout. That is, accept any advances you recorded for individual resistance exercises based on RPP and RPE only if your overall workout RPP is 2 or less and your overall workout RPE is 5 or less.

Avoid Bonking

Gating helps you avoid bonking, which is especially important in the advanced cardiolift where you work closer to the edge of the envelope. Bonking occurs when you deplete your main muscle fuel, glycogen. That is unlikely to occur at the beginning and intermediate levels, but two hours of continuous, high-intensity exercise—just a bit more than the advanced cardiolift described here—can deplete much of your internal glycogen. Among the earliest signs are unexpected fatigue and a corresponding inability to perform at the same level comfortably. That is followed progres-

---

* Each of the 8 unilateral exercises should take about 5 minutes (3 minutes of cardio, 2 minutes for setup, breakdown, and performance of three sets); the 4 ganged hip exercises should take about 12 minutes; and the triceps extension should require about 7 minutes; for a total of 59 minutes.

† Heat-up, 20 minutes; resistance exercises, including intermittent cardio-acceleration, 60 minutes; ROM cooldown, 10 minutes; for a total workout time of 90 minutes.

sively by an internal coldness and then shakiness. A general darkness ensues, which may be emotional—a pervasive gloom displaces the runner's high—and/or perceptually—everything actually looks gray. In a bonk this deep, your brain consumes 20 percent less glucose and 10–15 percent less oxygen. The heart races to unexpected heights, and the urge to sit or lie down becomes overpowering. Still more advanced stages of bonking include nausea, vomiting, and loss of consciousness.

Avoid bonking using body consciousness. Eating well is one key, particularly carbohydrate supplementation or carbo-loading. Have a good meal an hour before you work out, replete with low-glycemic (nonsugary) carbohydrates. Don't starve yourself before workouts under the mistaken impression that you will burn more fat that way. Depriving yourself of food before exercise is counterproductive to weight loss and exercise. As a further guard against bonking, you can consume 60 grams of carbohydrates (between 2 and 3 ounces) per hour of intense exercise, and have a good meal, such as a hearty sandwich, soon after your workout.

A second key to avoid bonking is to get plenty of sleep. I bonked twice last year, on both occasions following four rather than eight hours of sleep. Each instance started with an elevated heart rate—a sign of physiological distress. Similarly, two athletes in training returned from a spring vacation abroad and arrived in the gym sleepless for the preceding 24 hours, and both of their heart rates were 25 percent higher than usual. These experiences, and emerging scientific research, demonstrate the essential restorative power of sleep for exercise, and the hazards of exercising intensively without it (chapter 10). Eat and sleep well, and you should avoid bonking. If you feel it coming on anyway, stop your workout immediately and get something to eat, rest, and, if possible, take a nap. You should recover in a few hours.

Workout Logs

Written records of your workouts are always a matter of choice. Dispense with record keeping and cruise for a while now and then—it is a good way to add interest through variation, and simply enjoy your body. When you are building up to a high performance level, however, and particularly if you're a competitive athlete, maximizing your development is easier if you keep workout logs. Record keeping makes it easier to assess development over time, identify and break plateaus, and adjust workouts accordingly. Even if you are a recreational exerciser, keeping workout records provides invaluable feedback and helps motivate progress.

The IBC workout logs included in the appendix to this chapter, and available for download in 8½-by-11-inch format at www.MiracleWorkout.com (click on "Workout Logs"), accommodate the advanced IBC program. They include all the spaces you need to record the information to reach your peak performance goals in minimum time. At the advanced level, the IBC logs are designed to record numbers rather than qualitative indicators of RPP and RPE, so you will want to memorize those few corresponding numbers crucial to your decisions: 2 = weak, 3 = moderate, and 5 = strong. Once you have these firmly in mind, writing them down is easy.

Keeping workout logs may seem like a distraction, but they actually simplify your exercise routine, enabling you to record your RPP and RPE immediately following the third set of each resistance exercise and prescribe the weight and repetitions for your next workout. You will be surprised how relaxing and motivating it feels to have each workout prescribed fully when you first come into the gym, with no need for further decision and no room for wavering. And you may be amazed at how fast the human body responds to this stimulus.

Monitoring and Evaluating Your Progress

Evaluate your workout records periodically to guide your workouts intelligently—the mind–body connection in action again. The best way to follow workout progress is to display its parameters graphically (see figure 3.1, for instance), but that takes time and specialized software. You can learn a great deal from direct visual inspection of your cumulative workout logs—particularly if you circle each advance as described in the instructions for the advanced workout logs (appendix to this chapter). A quick glance down your workout log gives an immediate impression of your progress on a week-by-week basis. For the first few weeks of your advanced cardio-lift, you'll record five or six advances per workout, and on rare occasions you'll advance in every exercise. As diminishing returns set in, after perhaps two months of steady workouts, the advances decline to three or four and then one or two per workout. Then it's time to apply the plateau breakers described next.

Plateaus and Breakthroughs

After months of steady progress, every exerciser eventually enters a domain of diminishing returns, where progress in individual exercises or in overall workload slows or stops. Some muscle groups are more vulnerable to such plateaus than others. For most people, it's the arms and shoulders. Plateaus are inevitable as IBC brings you ever closer to your genetic limits. Along the way, however, pseudo-plateaus develop—plateaus that aren't real, and that you can crack with the right tools.

There are two dimensions to every plateau—mental and physical. I discovered the mental component some years ago by accident. I was stuck on the lat pull-down (figure 6.3, exercise 5), unable to advance for several weeks. One morning I inadvertently set the pin one plate heavier than the level where I was stuck, and completed the three sets without undue exertion and without noticing my error until I was finished. I had exposed a psychological barrier, and broken it by accident.

Based on that experience, I devised a more systematic way to break such psychological barriers. Reduce the number of repetitions to half your normal number or less, and do repeated sets of the exercise starting 10 percent below your plateau weight. Then add weight right up to and through your plateau. The very act of knowing you are lifting beyond your plateau weight registers in your subconscious, and sometimes that is all it takes to move to the next level. Your psychology adjusts, and the plateau dissolves—if it was indeed psychological. I have used this approach in training several athletes, and it has worked for some of them, too.

There is also a real physical barrier. You can never lift more weight, or do more repetitions, than your genetic potential enables you, and all the psychology in the world cannot break that kind of plateau. If the psychological approach fails, try the following physical technique to break a plateau. Do several different exercises involving the muscle or groups of muscles that have plateaued. Using the muscles in different neuromuscular coordination patterns recruit previously unused motor units, and create new levels of strength in the muscles as a whole. If your bench press is stuck, for example, do an inclined and reverse inclined bench press, in addition to using a flat bench, and throw in some pec flies, too. If the biceps are stuck, do a normal curl, a hammer curl, and other curls at different velocities. By shocking the muscles with these variations, you can add to your strength and break through plateaus that have not yet reached genetic limits.

Maxing

There is another way to break through plateaus—maxing. Every few weeks or whenever the spirit moves you, abandon your usual workout and do a maximal workout. Follow the heat-up with all the resistance exercises you normally do, but rather than three sets and the prescribed 8–12 repetitions, do one set of 6–10 repetitions using near-maximal weight—10–25 percent or more above your usual poundage, depending on the muscle group. You can alternate maxing with varying the range of motion and velocity of movement during each exercise, which recruits additional and new motor units, and harvests additional benefits in strength and power.

Maxing and velocity variation are reminiscent of the shock micro-cycles described in the older Soviet exercise literature. Maxing shocks the muscles, bones, ligaments, and nervous system like a dash of cold water in the face. The overload is a challenging workout—tackle it only when you're feeling strong—but the result is most satisfying. The very next workout may feel harder, but spurts of growth typically occur in a week or two following maxing. This technique has worked for a few athletes with whom I have tried it, although it hasn't been scientifically evaluated on a larger population. A similar method called overreaching enhances performance in resistance weight training. The next time you encounter a sustained plateau, you might try maxing and see how it works for you.

Maintenance and Periodization

Once you have reached your own self-defined level of peak performance, you will want to sustain it. Keeping a high level of physical fitness is easier than getting it in the first place. My physiology lets me sustain a reasonable level of fitness and performance with only one advanced cardiolift and two advanced cardio or cardiorom sessions per week. Such a minimal maintenance schedule requires just a few hours per week. A more aggressive maintenance schedule entails two cardiolift workouts per week plus one cardio session on any other day of the week.

IBC lends itself ideally to varying your exercise routine on macro- and microscales, or cross-training and periodization (chapter 4). Change exercises periodically, drawing from those illustrated in this book or from other sources. Cross-training and periodizing your workouts is your chance to be creative—it is fun, it keeps you in charge of your development, and is key to maintaining a healthy exercise routine for life. Periodization also enables you to reach higher levels and performance goals.

If you are an athlete, you may wish to taper—that is, to reduce your training as you approach your sport season. The purpose of tapering is to minimize negative impacts of training such as fatigue and glycogen depletion, while preserving the positive aspects like strength and endurance. If you continue IBC during your sport season, taper as you approach competitive events. Research shows that optimum tapering starts 4–28 days prior to competition, depending on your sport and workout routine. Tapering strategies that are most effective include maintaining training intensity, but reducing training volume (60–90 percent), and reducing workout frequency by no more than 20 percent. Although these tapering strategies improve performance by an average of only 3 percent, that small edge is often the difference between losing and winning.

Graduation

When you complete the advanced IBC program and progress steadily for a few months, you reach a level of fitness that you've probably never before attained. That feeling, you will discover, is its own reward. You may wonder where you can possibly go from here. The good news is you can go anywhere you want, and you will never exhaust the possibilities of Integrated Body Conditioning. Although it may seem like we have explored exercise comprehensively, there are many additional dimensions—power development, agility training, balance, plyometrics, specific sport skills—and they can all be incorporated into your IBC program. The excitement and satisfaction of learning and applying new approaches to the development of the human potential can easily occupy a lifetime. Consider spending, at most, six months of each year in the gym, and then cross-train with the outdoor IBC workouts detailed in the next chapter. Once you try those, and the home variations, you will fully appreciate the infinite possibilities of IBC.

Appendix to Chapter 6

Instructions for Use of Advanced Miracle Workout Logs

There are two different workout logs in the appendix to chapter 6, prescribed and generic. The prescribed workout log is based on the resistance exercises shown in figure 6.5, while the generic workout log is based on whatever resistance exercises you choose, plus the essential core (abdominal) exercises. The instructions for using the advanced workout logs are the same for both workouts, and almost identical to those for the intermediate workout logs described in the appendix to chapter 5.

There are two differences between the advanced and intermediate workout logs. First, the advanced logs are based on the Heart Rate Reserve (HRR) method described in chapter 6, rather than the HR_{MAX} method described in chapter 5. Second, the advanced logs are set up for recording Rating of Perceived Pain and Rating of Perceived Exertion using numerical scales introduced in chapter 6, rather than the verbal scales in chapter 5. With these two exceptions, follow the instructions in the appendix to chapter 5 for the advanced workout logs.

Advanced Miracle Workout Log, Cardiolift Phase, Prescribed

Name _____

CARDIOVASCULAR PARAMETERS AND HEART RATE TRAINING WINDOW

Active Rest _____ **BPM**   **Lower** _____ **BPM**   **Upper** _____ **BPM**   **Target** _____ **BPM**
(40 percent HRR)   (60 percent HRR)   (84 percent HRR)   (72 percent HRR)

WORKOUT# _____		WORKOUT# _____		WORKOUT# _____	
Date (m/d/y)	Day of Week	Date (m/d/y)	Day of Week	Date (m/d/y)	Day of Week

CARDIOVASCULAR CONDITIONING

Cardiovascular (Check)	Time (min)	Program	Level	KCals/ Av HR	Time (min)	Program	Level	KCals/ Av HR	Time (min)	Program	Level	KCals/ Av HR
Stair-Stepper ☐												
Treadmill ☐												
Cycle ☐												
Other ☐												

FREE WEIGHTS AND EXERCISE MACHINES

Exercise	wt, lbs	rep 8–12	sets (3)	RPP	RPE	wt, lbs	rep 8–12	sets (3)	RPP	RPE	wt, lbs	rep 8–12	sets (3)	RPP	RPE
1. Leg Press															
2. Leg Extension															
3. Leg Flexion															
4a. Hip Flexion															
4b. Hip Extension															

Exercise	wt, lbs	rep 8–12	sets (3)	RPP	RPE	wt, lbs	rep 8–12	sets (3)	RPP	RPE	wt, lbs	rep 8–12	sets (3)	RPP	RPE
4c. Hip Abduction															
4d. Hip Adduction															
5. Lat Pull-Downs															
6. Bench Press															
7. Overhead Press															
8. Arm Curls															
9. Triceps Extens.															
10. Core (Abs)															

OVERALL WORKOUT PARAMETERS

WinTim/Av. HR/Kcal	/ /	/ /	/ /
Weight Before/After	/	/	/
Water Used (liters)			
Workout RPP/RPE	/	/	/
Observations and Comments			

Advanced Miracle Workout Log, Cardiolift Phase, Generic

Name _____

CARDIOVASCULAR PARAMETERS AND HEART RATE TRAINING WINDOW

Active Rest _____ **BPM**   **Lower** _____ **BPM**   **Upper** _____ **BPM**   **Target** _____ **BPM**
(40 percent HRR)   **(60 percent HRR)**   **(84 percent HRR)**   **(72 percent HRR)**

WORKOUT# _____   WORKOUT# _____   WORKOUT# _____

Date (m/d/y)	Day of Week	Date (m/d/y)	Day of Week	Date (m/d/y)	Day of Week

CARDIOVASCULAR CONDITIONING

Cardiovascular (Check)	Time (min)	Program	Level	KCals/ Av HR	Time (min)	Program	Level	KCals/ Av HR	Time (min)	Program	Level	KCals/ Av HR
Stair-Stepper ☐												
Treadmill ☐												
Cycle ☐												
Other ☐												

FREE WEIGHTS AND EXERCISE MACHINES

Exercise (Write In)	wt, lbs	rep 8–12	sets (3)	RPP	RPE	wt, lbs	rep 8–12	sets (3)	RPP	RPE	wt, lbs	rep 8–12	sets (3)	RPP	RPE
1.															
2.															
3.															
4.															
5.															

Exercise	wt, lbs	rep 8–12	sets (3)	RPP	RPE	wt, lbs	rep 8–12	sets (3)	RPP	RPE	wt, lbs	rep 8–12	sets (3)	RPP	RPE
6.															
7.															
8.															
9.															
10.															
11.															
12.															

OVERALL WORKOUT PARAMETERS

WinTim/Av. HR/Kcal	/ /	/ /	/ /
Weight Before/After	/	/	/
Water Used (liters)			
Workout RPP/RPE	/	/	/
Observations and Comments			

Do not use this Workout Log without following the information and safety guidelines contained in the book *The Miracle Workout*. The Miracle Workout, and its agents, assume no liability for persons who use this Workout Log or change their exercise or physical activity. Copyright © 2002 by W. Jackson Davis. This Workout Log may be reproduced without change for personal use only.

Customize Your Miracle Workout

This section shows you how to adapt IBC to fit your unique needs and preferences. We begin by expanding on the gym workout to vary your IBC program with home, outdoor, and other options (chapter 7). Next we'll turn to exercise motivation—how to measure it, and how to keep it high (chapter 8). We will then see how IBC can work for special populations of exercisers (chapter 9), and wrap up with living the integrated life (chapter 10).

7

Do What You Love

Cross-training and periodization requires that you get out of the gym a few months each year. The variation keeps you fresh, interested, and exercising for the long haul, and helps bring you to your full genetic potential by countering physiological adaptation. IBC offers several possibilities for variation. Above all, the varied IBC workouts described in this chapter add fun to your IBC program and give you the means to customize your program to perfectly fit your exercise level, age, and preferences.

The Law of Specificity

The need for variety in exercise stems in part from the law of specificity. Specificity means that the training effect of any particular physical activity is specific to that activity, and does not transfer fully to other activities. Training one of your three energy systems, for example, doesn't transfer to the other two. This is one of the reasons that IBC is designed to condition all three of your energy systems in the same workout (chapter 2). Similarly, when you train on the leg press machine, the effect on your maximum jumping height is minimum, even though both movements involve the same energy systems—first and second gears—and the same muscles. The law of specificity governs even within individual exercises. Strength gains for any particular muscle or groups of muscles, for example, are specific to the exercise itself, the movement velocity, and even the range of movement or arc in which training takes place.

Specificity has implications for the transferability of gains. During a typical arm resistance exercise, the angular velocity around your elbow never exceeds 100 degrees per second. When a baseball pitcher throws, however, arm velocity measured about the elbow joint exceeds 700 degrees per second. Weightlifting therefore cannot prepare you fully for pitching a baseball, although it can help strengthen the foundation. Similarly, a soccer or football kick entails limb velocities up to 2,000 degrees per second, while typical limb velocities during resistance training in the gym are less than 10 percent of that. Such specificity implies that "the most effective way to train for a particular activity is to practice that activity regularly."[1]

You can do a simple self-experiment to observe the law of specificity in action. Train your aerobic system on a stationary cycle for a few weeks, and then move to the stair-stepper and see what happens. If you are like most people, you will feel like you are working and breathing unusually hard on the stair-stepper in comparison with the cycle, until your muscles and energy systems accommodate to the new activity after a few workouts. The same is true for any change in physical activity, in or out of the gym. Working hard in the garden does not necessarily improve your golf game, hiking does not necessarily improve your swimming performance, and cycling will not necessarily make you a better baseball batter.

Taken to its logical extreme, specificity might imply that whatever training effects you gain in the gym, you leave at the door when you exit—which is just as clearly untrue. You can disprove this logical extreme with another simple self-experiment. Before you start your IBC program, climb several flights of stairs, then measure your elapsed time, heart rate, and breathing frequency at the top. Then do IBC for a few weeks or months, and redo the same stair test, in the same amount of time. You'll feel the difference—less huffing and puffing, and a reduced heart rate response at the top, owing to the generalized physical conditioning attained with IBC.

This self-experiment illustrates an important qualifier to specificity—the central effects of training, those involving basic structural and functional changes, stay with you when you leave the gym to climb stairs, or venture onto the athletic field—anywhere, at home, work, and play. You also keep the toned body, the stronger and more enduring muscles, and the strengthened bones, ligaments, and tendons. The law of specificity evolved along with our hunter-gatherer ancestors. It worked well for them, assuring that their everyday activities prepared them optimally for the tasks required of them to survive. It also makes biological sense—we strengthen exactly the biological machinery that we use. Specificity throws a kink into modern exercise regimes, however. It means that if we commit narrowly to a particular type of exercise, such as weightlifting or flexibility training or jogging, we achieve only those training effects associated with that specific exercise. Specificity is partly why variety in exercise is so necessary to balanced development. Specificity is why IBC requires and adopts a full range of counterstrategies.

Variations on the IBC Theme

IBC is purposely comprehensive to maximize and generalize your conditioning, but the only way to achieve complete conditioning is to vary your IBC workouts. Cross-train and periodize to obtain the full benefits of different types of conditioning. Swimmers, for example, can cross-train by running, for a different challenge to the aerobic energy system. Dancers can train with resistance exercise and Range of Motion (ROM), an example of addressing two different energy systems. Golfers can cross-train by cycling, which will build endurance and strengthen hips—and so on.

Cross-train from the outset of your gym-based IBC program by varying cardio machines within and between every workout. Use the stair-stepper to cardio-accelerate before one resistance exercise, work the treadmill before the next, and jump rope before the third. Do your heat-up using the rowing machine in one workout, and the stationary cycle in the next. Such variety will recruit your full complement of motor units and provide the broadest possible cross-training of your energy systems, generalizing your cardiovascular conditioning.

Similarly, you can cross-train your joints in the cardiorom stage by learning and practicing a large range of basic ROM exercises. No two stretches or bends challenge any given joint in exactly the same way. Cross-train your muscles, bones, and ligaments in the cardiolift stage by working the same muscles or muscle groups using different exercise machines. Instead of doing only the bench press for your pecs, rotate or add inclined bench presses, bench barbell reach-overs, dumb-bell flies, and machine pec flies. Only by shocking your muscles with new patterns of movement can you use and build their full potential.

Certain muscles, such as the large-muscle groups of the lower body legs, have limited options. Two basic muscle groups, the extensors (quads) and flexors (hamstrings), for example, operate the knee. The bench squat is one of the best all-around exercises for these and a range of related muscles. Try it at different velocities to achieve a broader training effect. Alternate slow, even movements with more rapid, explosive ones that recruit larger motor units operated by bigger motor neurons. Cross-train these basic lower body muscles by alternating with machine exercises such as the leg press and other free-weight exercises like the dead lift. To minimize the risk of injury from these exercises, obtain instruction first from a certified trainer and use a spotter.

For a fun and educational approach to cross-training, learn every weight machine in your health club and then use as many as you can in any given period of a few months. After you master all the machines, move to exercises with free

Myth Buster 7: The Best Exercise Program

THE MYTH: There is a single workout that is best for everyone.

It would be nice if a single exercise program were perfect for everyone, but the law of specificity assures otherwise. Specificity means that the training effect from each exercise type, program, movement, and even velocity and range of movement is specific to the activity itself.

The implications can be astonishing. Research in the 1960s, for example, appeared to show a remarkable strength gain—5 percent per week—from static, or isometric, training, in which there is no movement, just contraction of your muscles against an external load. Subsequent research, however, showed that the gains were smaller and occurred predominantly for the exact joint angle used in training! Vary that angle just a few degrees, and there was no training effect.

There are as many best exercise programs as there are people with distinct exercise goals. Given the law of specificity and individual preferences, the best exercise depends on the training effect that you seek. If you want a flat belly, do the IBC workout for all-around conditioning, alternating with specialty abdominal workouts. To hit a baseball as hard as you can, do the foundational whole-body IBC workout in the off season, add sport-specific exercises, and spend plenty of time in the batter's cage.

If you seek the broadest, most comprehensive training of all of your energy systems and physiology that nature intended and enabled, IBC may be your best training approach. IBC systematically engages and conditions the full spectrum of human physiology (chapter 2), making it a sound all-around foundational training for any specific activity or sport. Then, when the foundation is strong, add specific exercises according to your individual goals.

THE REALITY: The best workout is the one that is tailored to your specific desired exercise outcomes and training effects.

The IBC Myth Buster

MYTH: There is one best exercise program.

FACT: The ideal program is IBC combined with exercises tailored to more specific goals.

weights—barbells and dumbbells. Unlike machine-based exercises, which are constrained to a one-size-fits-all model, free weights guarantee a workout customized to your particular anatomy and biomechanics. Free weights also require natural movements that engage all the muscles that operate any particular joint, and they typically work multiple joints as well as direct and indirect stabilizer muscles. The training effects from these more natural patterns of neuromuscular coordination transfer better to everyday life and athletics. The only downside of free weights is that using them properly requires more skill than machines, and the risk of injury may therefore be higher for inexperienced exercisers. Even when you have mastered free-weight exercises, however, after a few months it's time to leave the gym to explore other options—the outdoor IBC workouts.

Outdoor IBC Workouts

Outdoor IBC workouts not only provide essential exercise variety but are also the pinnacle of exercise pleasure and excitement. Just as common foods often taste best in a beautiful outdoor setting, outdoor exercise seems that much more invigorating. You can shift your IBC program outdoors for at least a quarter of every year, and even incorporate it into your vacations. To illustrate the possibilities, I will describe the beach IBC workout in some depth, and then extend the basic principles to other outdoor venues. This will give you the tools you need to design your own outdoor workout for wherever you live and whatever environment you love most.

The Beach IBC Workout

Of all the outdoor workouts, I have the most experience with the beach workout. It's also my favorite—there is something about the smell and feel of the ocean that interacts uniquely with exercise and the runner's high. The beach IBC workout we'll describe here assumes your cardiovascular system and joints are already well conditioned, and picks up at the cardiolift stage. Dry-sand power walking with a weighted backpack is the best and fastest cardio-driver and cardio-accelerator I have found. That's how I determine my maximum heart rate periodically to recalculate my heart rate training window (chapter 6) as my physical condition changes.

My beach workout begins at home, where I strap on my heart monitor and don my day pack. It is loaded with 40 pounds of PowerBlock portable dumbbells and 3 liters of water for a total weight of just under 50 pounds. I carry in hand the two 5-pound PowerBlock handles, each loaded with 5 pounds of weight, for the walk through the park to the beach with about one-third of my body weight in extra poundage. After a large drink of water, I am off. It takes 30 minutes at a brisk walking pace to reach the other end of the beach, just right for the heat-up. Weighted walking on dry sand while doing Nordic skiing movements with the handheld dumbbells is fantastic upper arm and shoulder work.

At the far end of the beach, I unload my backpack and take another long drink. The resistance component of the beach cardiolift now begins. There is no rule that says you have to limit yourself to any particular sequence or style of resistance exercise. The outdoor IBC workout offers an opportunity to transcend the relative rigidity of the gym workout. Try weighted forward lunges, or sideways lunges, or complex modern dance jumps and maneuvers with weight in hand. The guiding goal is variety in neuromuscular coordination pattern, and the only limit is your imagination.

As in the gym workout (chapters 4–6), the outdoor cardiolift continues with cardio-acceleration, followed by exercises that work the largest muscles. Squats are a great place to start. Set up your weights (adjust the PowerBlocks), walk or jog in the sand to cardio-accelerate into your heart rate training window, and then complete your first set of squats. Do as many sets as you like, up to four, with intermittent cardio-acceleration, then move to the next exercise—forward lunges, for example, with intermittent sand jogging for cardio-acceleration. Then try sideways lunges, which work the hips like no other exercise in or out of the gym, with intermittent cardio-acceleration, followed by toe raises for the ankles and lower legs (gastrocs). You get the pattern by now, which is already familiar from the gym workouts—just intersperse resistance exercises with intermittent cardio-acceleration while you watch the surf crash and listen to the seals bark.

Continue the beach cardiolift with upper body exercises. Alternate cardio-acceleration with sets of overhead presses, one-armed lat rows, push-ups, front, side, and back deltoid raises, shoulder shrugs, curls, and triceps extensions. You will find many of these exercises pictured in chapters 4–6. If you began your IBC program in the gym, you will be so familiar with resistance exercises that by the time you switch to outdoor workouts, you will be able to make informed selections from the hundreds of resistance exercises identified in various books on the subject—or just make up your own. Your PowerBlock portable dumbbells support almost any resistance exercise you can do in the gym. You can also use stretch tubing, which is lighter and easier to pack. As always, leave the core exercises—abdominal curls, for example, and dead lifts—for last, to keep the core as fresh as possible to the end.

Then, as always, complete your balanced beach workout with your ROM sequence. I generally do my ROMs without intermittent cardio-acceleration. I seldom use workout logs for outdoor workouts, though the generic logs in the appendices to chapters 4–6 would be suitable. Sometimes I leave the PowerBlock weights behind, carry only water and a picnic, and limit my beach workout to a cardiorom. In either case, the walk back home gives another 30 minutes of solid aerobic exercise and stunning scenery before a hot shower.

Other Outdoor IBC Workouts

The beach workout illustrates the general pattern for any outdoor IBC workout. I have used three other outdoor workouts: forest, river, and mountain biking. For the forest workout, I hike with a loaded backpack to some isolated glade for the cardiolift and ROM cooldown. At the advanced level, your heart is so strong that walking on flat ground, even with a weighted backpack, does not raise your heart rate into your training window, and jogging with so much weight is (for me) too much impact on the knees. I therefore climb for the heat-up, and walk or jog uphill and back to cardio-accelerate between resistance exercises. You could also cardio-accelerate by jumping rope, jogging in place, or calisthenics.

The river IBC workout is an antidote to the heat of summer. Pick a spot where the water runs clear and deep at an intermediate flow, and swim hard in place against the current for your heat-up and cardio-acceleration. Your heart rate monitor works fine in shallow water. Then step out onto the shore for your resistance and ROM exercises. I've done this water workout only in a river, although in principle it could be adapted to any body of water—lake or sea—swimming along the shore or out and back for your cardio-acceleration between resistance exercises.

I've done the outdoor workout in several locations using my mountain bike for the heat-up and cardio-acceleration. The same pattern is applicable in principle to any outdoor venue or activity—snowshoeing, Nordic skiing, cycling, what have you. Just warm up or heat up, cardio-accelerate between resistance exercises, and finish off with a ROM cooldown—all in the great out-of-doors. The outdoor IBC workouts are superb cross-training, sustaining the high level of conditioning you can reach in the gym, and they're great fun. You may even discover that your exercise niche is not the gym at all, but rather in the great outdoors.

The Home IBC Program

Maybe you already know that the gym is not your niche. Many first-time exercisers in particular find the gym an intimidating environment, and if that describes you, the home IBC program may be most suitable for starters. The three-step process is the same as described for the gym and outdoor IBC workouts—build up your cardiovascular system first, use that heart strength to power and sustain flexibility training, and then work in weightlifting. As in the gym and outdoor IBC workouts, you will experience little or no muscles soreness and the fastest development your genetics can support.

Implementing the home IBC program is a matter of deciding where in your home to exercise, how to cardio-drive and cardio-accelerate, and what resistance and ROM exercises to do. Your cardio options are varied. You can invest in a motorized cardio machine such as a treadmill for home use, but that requires space, the cost can be prohibitive, and you are then limited to a single cardio option. You may want to consider no-cost options that take no space at all, such as marching or jogging in place, jumping jacks, or stair climbing. Or you might consider inexpensive nonmotorized options, like a Bosu Ball, step-up box, or jump rope.

The Bosu Ball is loads of fun, although not the optimum beginning option because using it safely for cardio-acceleration requires intermediate or advanced agility and strength. The step-up box is a sturdy step or box of variable dimensions—12 by 14 by 18 inches is convenient for most people—or an adjustable platform. You can purchase a step-up box through many sporting goods stores, catalogs, and websites, or build your own from ½-inch plywood. To elevate your heart rate into your training window, step up onto the box like climbing onto a stair, and then step back off. Switch the leading foot regularly so you're not always stepping up with the same leg. Using a step-up box is a little like walking up stairs in place, and you will easily be able to reach and maintain the moderate- or vigorous-intensity heart rate target window you need for cardio-driving.

Whatever your choice for cardio-driving at home, you can use it for the warm-up or heat-up, and then alternate intermittent cardio-acceleration with resistance and/or ROM exercise. For resistance exercises, you can use the same equipment described for the outdoor IBC workouts—PowerBlock dumbbells or stretch tubing—and the same exercises. If you have more space at home and want to invest a few hundred dollars, you can purchase a new or used barbell and dumbbell weight set and bench that will provide a comprehensive full-body workout. If you choose the home workout as your primary conditioning program, you can vary your routine with home IBC workouts in the garden, patio or outdoors, as weather permits and the spirit moves you.

Let's assume you've chosen a step-up box for your first home beginning IBC workout. Place it wherever it is convenient to exercise—your bedroom, living room, in front of the TV, garage, patio—and simply climb on and off using a regular cadence. Breathe deeply and regularly as you exercise, and monitor your heart rate frequently. After your warm-up or heat-up, alternate cardio-acceleration with resistance exercises as described for the gym IBC workouts (chapters 4–6). Depending on your level, do one, two, or three sets of each resistance exercise (beginning, intermediate, and advanced levels, respectively) with interspersed cardio exercise. When you finish your resistance exercises, cool down with the same ROM sequences detailed in chapters 4–6, or your own custom selection. You have completed a comprehensive IBC workout, in the comfort and privacy of your own home.

The Lunchtime IBC Workout

Most of us work a sedentary day job, and even if your job is active, it may not provide adequate exercise. A recent study of 494 men showed that a high physical load in the workplace does not translate into higher physical fitness. The reason:

Physical activity performed at the workplace did not have adequate intensity, volume, and duration to effect positive changes in other motor and functional capacities.[2]

The day may come when all employers realize the benefits that employee fitness brings to the bottom line. Some employers, such as Sprint, have already seen the light, and developed an exercise-friendly workplace. Until others follow this lead, you may have to schedule your workouts around your job, either before or after—or during your lunch hour. The lunchtime IBC workout may be an option if you have an exercise facility close enough to your workplace. If your lunch break is an hour long, that leaves just 30 minutes for a workout, but that is time enough for a reasonable intermediate lower or upper body IBC workout, which you can alternate on sequential days. The prescription in figure 7.1 shows how it might work in a 30-minute exercise time block.

The lunchtime IBC workout in figure 7.1 will work your upper and lower body, as well as your core, and can accommodate the beginning- or intermediate-level IBC workout. When you graduate to the advanced level, you may need the extra time of one or two weekend workouts, where cardio and core could figure more prominently. If you don't have a gym near your workplace, consider an outdoor IBC workout over your lunch hour. And if you miss the social contact, recruit a workout partner.

FIGURE 7.1
THE LUNCHTIME IBC WORKOUT

The following schedule assumes you have a one-hour lunch break and can exercise for 30 continuous minutes during that time:

- **Monday.** Five-minute warm-up, 20-minute lower body workout, 5-minute ROM cooldown.

- **Tuesday.** Five-minute warm-up, 20-minute upper body workout, 5-minute ROM cooldown.

- **Wednesday.** Twenty-minute cardio, 10-minute core exercise and ROM cooldown.

- **Thursday.** Same as Monday.

- **Friday.** Same as Tuesday.

The Traveling IBC Workout

Job-related travel can disrupt an exercise routine, particularly if you do not have access to a gym when you travel. You can try booking hotels that have a gym—it is usually possible to find a block of time before or after work hours to keep your IBC program going despite professional travel. Even if you do not have access to a gym when you travel, though, you can do a hotel IBC workout with no equipment. Use normal calisthenics—jumping jacks or running in place—to cardio-drive, and use your body weight or stretch tubing for resistance exercises, concluded as always with your ROM cooldown. If you are on a short business trip—one week or less—two or three good cardiorom workouts will maintain your existing level of fitness and enable you to return to your home-based IBC program without backsliding too much. On a longer trip, include a weekly session of resistance exercises to minimize losses.

If you are at the intermediate exercise level, you can do an intermediate IBC workout in your hotel room by alternating rapid squats for aerobics, combined with resistance exercises such as toe raises, push-ups, partial abdominal curls, prone back arches, biceps curls (use a chair for weight), and triceps dips. You are again using your body weight for resistance, but these more difficult exercises will provide a suitable intermediate level of exercise. A more advanced IBC workout is difficult in a hotel room, but not impossible. You may prefer to use the opportunity to cross-train with long walks through the city or a run through a city park. At the very least, you can use business trips as an opportunity to sustain the fitness levels you have achieved at home by focusing on cardiorom and core exercises, which can sustain the foundation you bring back home.

Sport-Specific IBC Programs

The IBC program provides the ideal foundation for sport-specific training. In addition to the basic IBC workout, you need sport-specific exercises. You can use this three-step simple approach to prepare for any sport:

1. Use the advanced IBC workout (chapter 6) in the off season to build balanced physical capacities. That will strengthen your foundation, help minimize the risk of injury, develop mental strength and motivation, and prepare for skill development.
2. Identify the muscles and movements that are most important to your sport, and train those muscles using an integrated approach. Your coach or trainer can identify sport-specific muscle groups and exercises, and there are good books available on the topic.

3. Given the law of specificity, practice the sport itself, for both skill development and physical conditioning tailored to the sport.

Let's illustrate the three-step sport-specific approach with some examples drawn from popular sports.

Golf.

According to the traditional view, golf is not a vigorous sport, which has led to the misconception that physical conditioning is not as important for golfers. Tiger Woods's conditioning regimen, which includes hard resistance training, has helped dispel that myth. You are more likely a recreational golfer who simply wants to increase the quality and enjoyment of your game, and of course shave a few strokes off the bottom line. If you currently are in less-than-perfect physical condition, you may be dragging by the 18th hole. If you could feel as fresh at the end as you did at the beginning, it would improve both your score and your fun.

Start with the first step above: general and balanced body conditioning using IBC at whatever level is appropriate to your starting physical condition. That will train your energy systems and provide a sound general foundation for golf-specific exercises. Then learn the muscles and joints that are critical to your golf game, and the exercises to develop them. They include particularly the wrists, arms, and shoulders, but golf also demands hip and trunk flexibility, and core strength for the swing. Recent research has emphasized the special importance of hip strength for better golf scores. To avoid overuse injuries such as stress fractures of the ribs, strengthen those shoulder muscles. And don't neglect the legs—the swing puts significant torque on both knees, during both the takeaway and follow-through, but particularly during the downswing and as your weight shifts to the leading leg at the end of the swing.

To continue your physical preparation for golf, add resistance and ROM exercises to your foundational IBC workout to condition golf-specific muscles and joints on both sides of your body. You can either extend your normal IBC workout with these specialty exercises or create a new golf-specific workout that you alternate with the foundational workout. To complete your golf-specific preparation, practice at the driving range. You need that time not only to counter specificity, but also for the skill development that will make your game shine. When you get to the links on game day, don't neglect a pre-play warm-up and stretching. Research shows that a warm-up will improve your game and cut your chance of injury by half.

Soccer.

Use the same general approach to ready yourself or your team for any sport. Soccer, for example, traditionally emphasizes the lower body. We've used the advanced

IBC program for off-season foundational conditioning, which can be combined with soccer-specific exercises such as hip abduction and adduction to strengthen lateral and scissors kicks. Add sideways lunges and other sport-related moves with weights in hand to bring sport-specific plyometrics to bear, and merge these with aerobics and ROM to create a fully integrated soccer workout. Do all of the sport-specific conditioning over a wide range of movement velocities to maximize transferability from the gym to the field. Don't neglect the upper body, which among other things is essential in soccer for contesting the ball.

Any Sport.

Perhaps you are a recreational or competitive swimmer. Supplement the foundational IBC workout with stroke-specific upper body muscle conditioning. Are you a tennis buff? Bob Hansen, a Hall of Fame tennis player, has used IBC to strengthen his already awesome serve and to train national-caliber players. The general approach to these sports, and indeed to any sport, is the same as for golf and soccer detailed above. Identify the muscles, joints, and movements involved in the sport and train them at elevated heart rates. Employ range and velocity variation to mimic movement velocities in the sport. Combine this with the full-body IBC workout off-season as your foundation, and plenty of practice at the sport itself, and watch your individual capacities and team performance soar.

IBC and Other Exercise Systems

If you already have an exercise program going that works for you, stick with it. You can make some small modifications that will provide the additional benefits of IBC. If your current exercise program already has you in good cardio and ROM shape, you need only add cardio-acceleration to your current program and do it at an elevated heart rate. If your current program does not entail cardio or ROM exercise, prepare yourself by going through the cardio and cardiorom phases of IBC at the appropriate level.

We have integrated IBC with plyometrics, for example, to train athletes. Plyometrics is an advanced exercise method that takes advantage of stretching a muscle, which causes a reflexive contraction that adds to a voluntary command to produce a supercontraction. We've incorporated it with IBC for cardio-acceleration between resistance exercises. Plyometrics is extremely effective for athletes, and can be fashioned into sport-specific moves such as volleyball spikes or basketball jump shots and footwork in combination with a step-up box for agility training. Plyometrics are relatively high impact on joints, however, and most appropriate as specialty power training for younger exercisers and advanced, well-conditioned athletes.

Eastern exercise systems such as Yoga and the martial arts may be the oldest, most comprehensive, all-around exercise mind–body approaches ever practiced. They combine a wide range of positions and movement velocities with natural, multijoint exercises to create a disciplined and balanced approach to conditioning. Some martial arts already have aerobic components, while others can be very slow and deliberate. Yoga is a case in point. It has a popular reputation as a meditative practice, which it is, but certain forms are as physically demanding as any exercise. In her book *Power Yoga,* Beryl Bender Birch describes just such a dynamic exercise approach, based on the integration of Yoga with aerobics, and identifies the heat-up as the first axiom of what she calls the Power Yoga Workout. Such combinations of yoga or the traditional martial arts with cardio-acceleration may be among the most balanced and comprehensive exercises you can do.

The variations on the IBC theme are infinite, as you may be starting to appreciate. Any sport, movement, or exercise system becomes integrated exercise if you combine it with the basic principles and practices of IBC—integrate exercises, do them at an elevated heart rate, and progress based on biofeedback. These combinations, indoor and out, can add variety and fun to any exercise program, and when you do what you love, you will do it best.

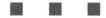

8

Stay in the Game

Perhaps you have noticed that in the first week of every year, the gym overflows with enthusiastic exercisers, while by the end of February you have it to yourself. What happened to those New Year's resolutions, and how can you keep your own exercise resolution from dissolving? The biggest challenge of any exercise program, including IBC, is not getting it started, but keeping it going. IBC makes staying in the exercise game easier, because there are so many rewarding variations. IBC still requires organization and discipline, and at advanced levels it is hard work. This chapter illuminates the demotivation demons and shows you how to deflect them in advance, and recover quickly if they get the better of you.

How Bad Do You Want It?

In exercise, sports, and life, motivation is the key ingredient. There is a simple way to estimate your own motivation for exercise. Fill out the exercise motivation questionnaire below (figure 8.1) and add up your score. Then we'll discuss what it means.

Scores on this motivation questionnaire range from 7 to 35. High scores signify greater motivation to exercise, while a score lower than 24 suggests that the motivational tools discussed in this chapter may have immediate relevance. Even if you scored above 24, though, you still need these tools. Elite athletes experience motivational ups and downs, and for the rest of us, the road to deconditioning is paved with the best intentions. The best way to avoid a relapse in your exercise pro-

FIGURE 8.1
EXERCISE MOTIVATION QUESTIONNAIRE

The purpose of this questionnaire is to estimate your motivation to exercise. Check the box corresponding to the alternative that fits you best.

	Extremely uncharacteristic	Somewhat uncharacteristic	Neither characteristic nor uncharacteristic	Somewhat characteristic	Extremely characteristic
1. I don't get discouraged easily.	☐	☐	☐	☐	☐
2. I work harder than I have to.	☐	☐	☐	☐	☐
3. I seldom if ever let myself down.	☐	☐	☐	☐	☐
4. I'm the goal-setting type.	☐	☐	☐	☐	☐
5. I'm good at keeping promises, especially the ones I make to myself.	☐	☐	☐	☐	☐
6. I impose much structure on my activities.	☐	☐	☐	☐	☐
7. I have a very hard-driving, aggressive personality.	☐	☐	☐	☐	☐
SCORING SCALE	**1**	**2**	**3**	**4**	**5**

Directions: After you have checked each box, score it according to the scoring scale marked below the last set of boxes, and then add your total score for all seven questions.

Adapted from R. K. Dishman, W. Ickes, and W. P. Morgan, "Self Motivation and Adherence to Habitual Physical Activity." Printed with permission from *J. Appl Soc Psychol* 10 (1980), pp. 115–132. Copyright © V. H. Winston & Son, Inc. All rights reserved. Subsequently published in H. B. Falls, A. M. Baylor, and R. K. Dishman, *Essentials of Fitness* (Philadelphia: Saunders, 1980), pp. 263–265.

gram is to understand your own behavior and attitudes toward exercise, and the best place to start is to know your stage of exercise. As you read the five stages below, see if you can identify your stage, and we'll discuss what it means.

The Stages of Exercise

The first stage of exercise is pre-contemplation, a big term for a simple idea. This stage pertains to people who are not yet ready to make a commitment to exercise.

If you're in this stage, you are not even thinking about exercise. People in this first stage are maintaining the status quo. That cannot be you, because you have already read this far. You are clearly thinking about it, and at least in the process of making a commitment.

The second stage of exercise is contemplation. Here exercise has your attention, but not yet your commitment. You are a ripe plum, and need just a nudge to get your exercise program under way. This nudge can come from inside or out, and take one of two forms: the carrot or the stick. The carrot is the reward of exercise—health and wellness for example, or knowing you have a great body. The stick is the real or potential punishment of not exercising—the risk of illness, for example, or being overweight. You could be in this contemplation stage—that would be consistent with your reading this far. But we think you are further along the path.

Preparation is the third stage of exercise. The feeling at this stage is easy to recognize—you are pumped up at the prospect of getting your exercise program under way, and ready to go. Motivation can be like a switch with just two positions—off and on. As the philosopher Franz Kafka wrote,

> From a certain point onward, there is no longer any turning back. That
> is the point that must be reached.[1]

In the preparation stage, your switch is on. You have reached Kafka's point of no return. You may even be doing some kind of physical activity already, although by definition it is less than the minimum recommended by health and exercise professionals to reap the health benefits of exercise, and it's not enough to satisfy your growing drive.

The minimum amount of exercise that confers measurable benefits, according to the U.S. surgeon general, is 30 minutes of moderate physical activity, accumulated over the whole day, for three to five days a week. If you take a brisk 15-minute walk twice a day, for example, you are exercising at that minimum. The American College of Sports Medicine (ACSM) defines the minimum as vigorous exercise for 20 minutes at least three days a week, noting that the two standards are part of a continuum. You get as much benefit from a little vigorous exercise as you do from a larger volume of moderate exercise.

The National Academy of Sciences (NAS), the agency that establishes nutrient intake recommendations for the United States and Canada, changed these exercise standards in 2002. The massive NAS report, available online (www.nap.edu), significantly revises the conventional wisdom about both diet and exercise. Regarding physical activity, the NAS report indicated that

. . . some benefits can be achieved with a minimum of 30 minutes of moderate intensity physical activity most days of the week. However, 30 minutes per day of regular activity is insufficient to maintain body weight in adults in the recommended body mass index range from 18.5 up to 25 kg/m² and achieve all the identified health benefits fully.[2]

That is, the NAS considers the surgeon general's earlier recommendation for 30 minutes a day of moderate exercise as a minimum consistent with health and wellness, but not sufficient to keep the pounds off. The NAS report established the following new standard for appropriate levels of physical activity:

. . . to prevent weight gain as well as to accrue additional, weight-independent health benefits of physical activity, 60 minutes of daily moderate intensity physical activity (e.g., walking/jogging at 4 to 5 mph) is recommended. . . . For children, the physical activity recommendation is also 60 minutes or more of daily activity and exercise.[3]

An hour a day keeps the pounds away. That new standard may surprise you, particularly if you have read or heard about exercise programs that promise benefits in just a few minutes of exercise a day. Unfortunately, those mini programs represent wishful thinking. They can't increase your health and wellness measurably, and they are inadequate for weight management, because they simply don't add up to enough exercise volume. They may nonetheless help motivate to start a more comprehensive and beneficial exercise program, schedule a regular exercise time, and enjoy the process. If you are not already in the preparation stage of exercise, these mini programs can help you get there.

I think you are in the preparation stage already, but you could have passed beyond it and be among the 11 percent of Americans who already exercise regularly. In that case, you have entered the action stage. In this fourth stage of exercise, you are meeting the surgeon general's minimum exercise standard of 30 minutes of moderate exercise a day three to five days each week, but you have been exercising at this level for less than six continuous months. According to sports psychologists, the brief tenure of your exercise career makes you more vulnerable to relapse. Even if you are in the action stage, and even if you have been an exerciser all your life, a relapse to inactivity is a continuous threat that requires vigilance and skill to avoid. Like life itself, staying with any exercise program can be an unremitting challenge.

Maintenance is the fifth stage of exercise readiness. That's when you have been exercising at the surgeon general's minimum level of 30 minutes of moderate exercise three to five days per week for at least six continuous months. It may feel that you have arrived. Arrival, however, is a daily requirement, and if you don't meet the challenge, deconditioning is astonishingly rapid. Cardiovascular conditioning fades in days, muscle strength wanes in weeks, and bone and ligament strength disappears in months. Your body wants to know, *What have you done for me lately?* Your task is to design your exercise program so you come up with a good answer at least three times a week. It is possible to achieve a lifetime commitment to exercise if you recognize and deflect the exercise demotivation demons.

The Demotivation Demons

Dropout rates from voluntary fitness and exercise programs range from 9 to 87 percent, with an average of 45 percent. Remarkably, the dropout rate among almost 4,000 cardiac patients in 14 different studies was similar—about half quit. You might think that people recovering from heart attacks would be less prone to drop out of an exercise program, but research shows instead that exercise motivation is fickle even when the stakes are high. Without proper tools and support, people are dropout prone regardless of the risk. In contrast, cardiac patients who received instruction in motivational tools and then practiced them had a dropout rate of only 12 percent, most for unavoidable family emergencies. What is required, in addition to your IBC program, is an ongoing exercise in the mind–body connection that keeps your commitment high.

The largest single reason people give for avoiding exercise is, according to the American College of Sports Medicine, lack of time. This is an unfortunate myth, for while exercise unquestionably takes time, it gives back far more. In the short term, you will sleep more soundly, and you may need less, leaving more time for waking life. The discipline and organization of IBC carries over to the rest of your life. When combined with the conditioning of your three energy systems, your waking hours can become more efficient and productive, creating more time for everything.

In the longer term, research shows that exercise capacity is the single most predictive indicator of longevity. The longevity data suggest that every one hour you spend in vigorous exercise adds seven high-quality hours to your life. That is a remarkable investment ratio, and it adds up to a startling conclusion. Start IBC at age 40 and do it three times a week for the rest of your life and you may add nearly 2.5 high-quality years to a life expectancy of 76 years—not to mention the satisfaction you'll get from being fit. If you start as a teenager, you can add at least five years to your life and vastly increase your quality of life.

Regular exercise can even spare you time in a hospital or nursing home. Thank goodness they are there when we need them, but no one wants to spend time in a hospital or nursing home if they can help it. In fact, hospital stays represent one of the riskiest things we can do. Recent research shows that 190,000 Americans die in hospitals each year from causes unrelated to their visit. That's more than four times the risk of fatality than the next most dangerous routine activity, driving a car.

Myth Buster 8: Too Much Time

THE MYTH: Exercise takes too much time. Already I don't have enough time to get through each day.

Only 11 percent of U.S. citizens exercise regularly. Ask the other 89 percent why they don't, and the first answer you're likely to hear is that they don't have enough time. And it is certainly true that in this busy world, we barely have time to survive and still maintain relationships with ourselves, friends, and family. How can we justify, to ourselves and to others, the "additional" time that exercise programs appear to require? This perceived lack of time can be a program buster for any exercise regime, not just IBC.

There is no denying that exercise takes a time commitment. Depending on your goals and motivation, you can spend two, six, or more hours a week doing IBC. Once you get rolling, however—in just a few short weeks—you'll find that you work far more efficiently at everything else each day, creating more time for everything. You'll sleep more soundly, and may need less sleep each night to feel great the next day. From this perspective alone, IBC may at least break even when weighed on the scale of time.

It is the long-term time savings, however, that is the clincher. A study carried out at Stanford University and the Veterans Affairs Palo Alto Health Care System and published in March 2002 in the *New England Journal of Medicine* concluded that your physical fitness level is the best single predictor of how long you will live. It is more important even than smoking habits, blood pressure level, or your family history of heart attacks. People who exercise regularly live much longer, and their quality of life is much higher.

One of the authors of the study, Dr. J. Edwin Atwood, put it as directly as it gets: "If you exercise and improve your exercise capacity, you will increase your longevity." Rita Redberg, spokesperson for the American Heart Association, said, "Exercise is the fountain of youth. . . . It will save your life." The message is clear. Survival truly is of the fittest! Exercise doesn't take time, it gives time, by providing both a longer day and a longer, better life.

THE REALITY: IBC gives more net time for everything, and increases the quality of life, too.

The IBC Myth Buster

MYTH: Exercise takes too much time.

FACT: IBC gives you far more time than it takes.

After fully grasping the implications of exercise, and incorporating it into a belief system and lifestyle, many people go through a metamorphosis. Part of that change is that you understand deep down in your bones that exercise does not take time; it gives you time, and lots of it. This transformed perspective puts exercise in a different light, elevating it from an optional activity you do if you can spare the time, to an essential activity that you know will give you even more time on every level (see p. 178).

As a first step, learn and heed the dropout indicators. The American College of Sports Medicine divides predictors of exercise dropout into three categories: personal, program, and other (figure 8.2). As you read these predictors, see if you can identify any present in you, and then we'll see how to deal with them.

FIGURE 8.2
EXERCISE DEMOTIVATION DEMONS

1. Personal Variables

Primary (most predictive)

Cigarette smoking

Inactive leisure time

Sedentary occupation

Blue-collar occupation

Overweight or obese

Depressed

Secondary (less predictive)

Age and gender

Personality factors

Educational attainment

Poor credit rating

2. Program Variables

Inconvenient time or location

Excessive cost

Lack of exercise variety

Exercising alone

Lack of reinforcement

Inflexible exercise goals

Low enjoyment

Poor program leadership

3. Other Variables

Lack of spouse support

Excessive job travel

Injury

Change of job

Change of residence

Inclement weather

From American College of Sports Medicine, *ACSM's Guidelines for Exercise Testing and Prescription*, sixth edition (Philadelphia: Lippincott Williams & Wilkins, 2000), box 12.1, p. 239. Original source: B. A. Franklin, "Program Factors That Influence Exercise Adherence: Practical Adherence Skills for Clinical Staff," in R. Dishman (editor), *Exercise Adherence: Its Impact on Public Health* (Champaign, IL: Human Kinetics, 1988), pp. 237–258. Copyright © 2000 by American College of Sports Medicine. Reproduced by permission of Lippincott Williams & Wilkins.

Personal dropout predictors include four key variables: cigarette smoking, inactive leisure time, a sedentary occupation, and blue-collar employment. Cigarette smoking is the most predictive, based on research on cardiac patients. When that was the only variable present, the dropout rate in one series of studies was 59 percent. When the remaining three of these key variables were also present, the dropout rate zoomed to 95 percent. All four of these demotivation demons are behavioral variables—that means you're the boss, you control them. It's hard, granted, but you can quit smoking, and you can increase physical activity in your leisure time. Switching jobs may be harder, but if you have a sedentary job, you may be able to add some movement to it, or do the lunchtime IBC workout (chapter 7).

Next on the list of personal variables that predict exercise dropout is body weight—or, rather, too much of it. Heavier people are less physically active, and less motivated to start and continue with an exercise program. In one study of 269 obese men and women, more than 90 percent missed at least two-thirds of the scheduled exercise sessions. The reasons may be physical—the greater challenge of doing any activity when you are overweight—or psychological—dissatisfaction with body image and consequent avoidance of group exercise. Anyone who is or has been overweight understands the double bind only too well. You become less motivated to undertake the very activity—exercise—that can reduce your body weight. This classic chicken-and-egg conundrum has a solution. Master the motivational tools in the paragraphs below, practice them daily, and commit to doing this for the rest of your life.

Depression presents another chicken-and-egg dilemma. According to the American Psychological Association, exercise helps clinically depressed people beat the blues, perhaps because of the release of endorphins we discussed earlier in connection with the runner's high. The dilemma arises because although exercise reduces depression, depression itself reduces the motivation to exercise. Even one good exercise session can begin to ameliorate some of the symptoms of mild depression. If you have a friend or loved one who suffers from depression, introduce them to IBC, help get them started, and see what happens.

Gender also influences exercise participation and dropout. Women generally do less vigorous physical activity, particularly when they are younger. The differences in physical activity are cultural rather than biological, and therefore easier to change. Social structures and constraints have in the past presented females with fewer opportunities to engage in exercise. That is changing, reflected by legislation such as Title IX, which guarantees equal gender access to sports and physical activity. The biological reality is that women are just as capable of hard exercise as men, they show similar physiological responses to exercise, and they benefit equally or even more. Females may experience a higher risk of certain sports-related injuries, however, and require special precautions when exercising during pregnancy (chapter 9).

Age is also associated with less physical activity, although the increasing number of seniors in top physical condition belies that cultural stereotype, too. For many and perhaps most people, there is no physiological reason not to exercise vigorously right up to the end of life. You can expect certain biological changes no matter how hard you exercise, of course, but that doesn't mean you can't stay in good physical shape. There is even a term for it: the rectangularization of the aging process. Instead of reaching a peak in your 20s and resigning yourself to steady decline thereafter, you hold that peak as long as you can, or at least slow the rate of decline, so the trajectory of your physical condition over time looks like a rectangle instead of a bell. Seniors should also follow certain special precautions prior to and during exercise (chapter 9).

Demotivation demons also include characteristics of your exercise program. At the top of this list is inconvenient time or location. IBC can resolve convenience issues easily—you can work out whenever and wherever you want. You still have to carve out the time from a busy schedule, but most people can find at least a couple of hours per week for IBC. That's the equivalent of just one or two television programs. You do not even have to miss those programs if you set up your home IBC workout (chapter 7) in front of the tube, although make sure that the distraction of television does not cause your exercise form to deteriorate. Sports fans, you can do a complete beginning home workout, or a thorough core workout, while watching a televised sports event.* It can be a fun group activity, and you and your friends may feel better about watching those televised games if you are simultaneously improving your health.

After time, excessive cost is a close second to inconvenience on the list of program demotivation demons. IBC may provide the best possible solution to the cost factor. The home IBC workout is inexpensive and requires minimum equipment. Gym memberships do cost money, but you can shop carefully for bargains and often find family memberships. Above all, IBC does not cost net money—as in the case of time, IBC saves more than it costs. IBC is cost effective, in the terminology of health professionals, in the sense that it reduces several risks at the same time, and therefore saves far more than it costs (see the sidebar in chapter 4).

Dropout-prone behavior is also associated with program variables such as lack of variety, solitariness, lack of reinforcement, inflexible goals, poor program leadership, and lack of enjoyment. IBC systematically and purposefully dispels every

---

* Don't mix TV or any other distraction with an intermediate or advanced IBC workout, however, because concentration on form is an essential safety requirement at higher exercise levels.

one of these demotivation demons. The variety of IBC options is as infinite as movement itself, and includes gym (chapters 4–6), home, and outdoor workouts (chapter 7), as well as cross-training and periodization over the year to keep your program dynamic and interesting. IBC is amenable to partner or group workouts, which can multiply the fun. IBC builds reinforcement—reward—into your exercise program from the start, and its goals are as flexible as you. Program leadership can be in your own hands, and for most people who do IBC, it is the most enjoyable physical activity since child's play.

The third category of demotivation demons identified by the American College of Sports Medicine is termed "other variables." This broad but important category includes the lack of support by spouses or peers, but also excessive job travel, injury, job change or move, and even inclement weather. Spousal and peer support are crucial—in one study of men, the dropout rate from an exercise program was 20 percent if their partner was supportive, but 60 percent if the spouse was unsupportive. The message: Keep your significant other involved, perhaps even as your workout partner.

Continuing with the demons of figure 8.2, excessive job travel can disrupt exercise, but you can counter it with traveling IBC workouts (chapter 7). Reducing the risk of injury is one of IBC's strongest suits; we have never experienced an injury attributable to the workout itself. Job change and moves disrupt exercise routines, but they are temporary and you can reestablish your IBC program as soon as you get settled. Inclement weather—now, there at last is something that IBC can't affect! On the other hand, the gym is a climate-controlled environment, and the beach IBC workout (chapter 7) in the rain or fog can be a beautiful thing—and you generally have the shore all to yourself.

Deflating the Demons

There are two complementary approaches to defeat the exercise demotivation demons: reactive and preventive. The reactive approach entails waiting until the dropout behavior occurs and then reversing it. The preventive approach defeats dropout behavior before it starts, and is therefore more effective. A simple method to implement the preventive approach is the learn–heed–change process (figure 8.3). Learn the dropout predictors summarized in the preceding section (figure 8.2); heed them in yourself by taking personal inventory; and when you find the demons, celebrate! You just took the essential first step to exorcise the demotivation demon. Only now can you change your behavior and its underlying cause, your belief structure.

Take a few minutes now to go through the list of dropout indicators and see whether any apply to you. When you find matches, consider ways you can change the behavior or the belief. You're well on your way to defeating dropout behavior.

FIGURE 8.3
THE THREE-STEP PROCESS FOR EXORCISING DEMOTIVATION DEMONS

Follow this "learn–heed–change" process to prevent exercise dropout:

1. **Learn the predictors.** The first step is to learn and understand the variables that make people dropout prone. Figure 8.2 summarizes them for you.

2. **Heed them in yourself.** The second step is to undertake a personal inventory to see if any of the dropout indicators characterize your behavior or beliefs. You have to identify your demons before you can exorcise them.

3. **Change.** The third step is to dispel your demotivation demons. Change your behavior or your beliefs, or devise strategies to work around them. Figure 8.4 is your tool kit to implement this change.

Regardless of how pumped up you feel right now about exercise in general and IBC in particular, maintaining a lifetime of healthy exercise habits will eventually require that you master the full arsenal of motivational tools. I know this from personal experience; I have needed nearly every one of the tools at one time or another, and I know you will benefit from them, too. These tools, all of which exercise the mind–body connection, will help you defeat the demotivation demons. They begin with the motive force behind all learned human behavior—beliefs.

Believe in Yourself

Beliefs are learned associations about cause and effect. You learned from your experiences that when A occurs, B follows. Or when you do X, Y happens. Those associations stick in your brain as a "belief," and help tint your perceptual lenses to that special hue through which you observe and interpret the world. Many beliefs, and perhaps most, originate in childhood. Girls from earlier generations, for example, learned early in life that exercise was unfeminine, and often suffered social humiliation and exclusion by peers. The behavior (exercise or physical activity) caused social pain (negative reinforcement), and the resulting learned belief (*I should avoid exercise because it is unfeminine*) spared the child further punishment—a useful defense mechanism for the budding prepubertal personality.

Many beliefs formed in childhood become useless or harmful in adulthood.

The belief that exercise was unfeminine may have spared the girl of yesteryear social pain in youth, but it also worked against her best interests as a young woman and adult. We know now that exercise is the best antidote for the three greatest causes of morbidity and mortality in women—osteoporosis, breast cancer, and heart disease. The good news is that you can discard or change outmoded or counterproductive beliefs. All that belief baggage resides in our brains in physical form, embedded in networks of nerve cells, and if you can just make the corresponding belief conscious, you can yourself rewire those neural networks, using the three-stage change process of Figure 8.3.

The IBC Myth Busters can help identify and dispel the beliefs that betray exercise. The Myth Busters replace destructive beliefs with new and more accurate beliefs that support your IBC program. The Myth Busters are therefore a systematic way to support the three-stage change process. Think of them as "debugging" devices that literally help change your mind.

Build Self-Efficacy

Simple beliefs aggregate into larger complexes that collectively create our picture of the world and our place in it, including the ability to influence for the better our environment and fate, or our self-efficacy. Self-efficacy is an example of a meta-belief, a complex of smaller beliefs that together determine your self-image, confidence, and capacity to control and direct your life. Exercise professionals identify self-efficacy as one of the best predictors of the success of an exercise program. The American College of Sports Medicine suggests a simple test of your self-efficacy. Just answer this question: On a scale of 0 to 100, how confident are you that you can change your behavior for the better? Take a moment now to think about it, and jot down your answer.

Do you have your self-efficacy score? According to the ACSM, if you estimated your self-efficacy as 70 percent or above, you have a good chance of making a behavioral change successfully, such as getting your IBC program started and keeping it going. If your estimate of your self-efficacy is below 70 percent, direct your energy toward reinvigorating and updating your belief system. Identify those meta-beliefs that stand in the way of greater self-efficacy, and those specific beliefs that interfere with your exercise program. You cannot jump belief barriers until you see them clearly, but once you do, the next step is easier. The catch-22 here is that you need a certain amount of self-efficacy just to get this process started in the first place. You need a motivation tool kit.

Your Motivation Tool Kit

A wide variety of tools is available to help manage and sustain exercise motivation (figure 8.4). At one time or another, typically sooner rather than later, we all need

FIGURE 8.4
YOUR MOTIVATION TOOL KIT

Exercise psychologists suggest a dozen motivational methods to help initiate and maintain your exercise program. They are:

1. **Preparing.** Establish realistic expectations.

2. **Shaping.** Start low and build steadily as you go.

3. **Goal setting.** Individualize your goals based on your preferences.

4. **Reinforcement.** Know what turns you on, and use it.

5. **Stimulus control.** Create environmental cues that stimulate you to exercise.

6. **Contracting.** Make agreements to support your exercise program.

7. **Cognitive strategies.** Create intentional plans to keep you exercising.

8. **Social support.** Enlist support from others to keep you exercising.

9. **Self-management.** Be your own behavioral therapist.

10. **Relapse prevention.** Develop strategies to deal with exercise relapses.

11. **Relapse recovery.** Do not beat up on yourself—get back in the saddle!

12. **Generalization training.** Make physical activity a way of life.

Adapted from American College of Sports Medicine, *ACSM's Guidelines for Exercise Testing and Prescription,* sixth edition (Philadelphia: Lippincott Williams & Wilkins, 2000), box 12.3, p. 243. Copyright © 2000 by American College of Sports Medicine. Reproduced by permission of Lippincott Williams & Wilkins.

them. Let's assemble all the tools here, in one kit, so you will always have them handy and never have to succumb to the demotivation demons.

Your first tool is preparing. Start by making sure your expectations for exercise are realistic. Exercise professionals even recommend setting your initial expectations low, because the likelihood of achieving them is higher, and achievement is motivating. Exercise is a journey, not a destination, and the first priority is just to get that journey started. At the beginning level of IBC, the lowest expectations you can entertain include feeling better, lowering health costs, and living longer—not a bad return for your investment.

Your motivation tool kit continues with shaping—a tried-and-true psychological technique that means that you keep increasing your expectations and goals as you progress. You shape your goals to your constantly improving physical and mental condition. Shaping helps preserve that fresh feeling of doing something new, so your growth and development become self-perpetuating. The IBC method of progression is an example of shaping—it increases your exercise workload in direct proportion to your self-assessed capacity, in accord with how you feel (chapters 4–6).

An example illustrates how you might be able to use shaping for weight management. Overweight people are sometimes hesitant to exercise in a group situation. One shaping strategy is incremental exposure. Start your exercise program alone, and then later, at the next level of shaping, get a workout partner. When you are comfortable working out with a partner, expand your exposure by joining a larger group, for brief times at first, followed by longer periods and then full workouts. Such an approach is effective in sustaining exercise for people of normal weight, and it could work for overweight people, too.

Shaping works hand in hand with another tool in your kit, goal setting. Goals represent one of the most important organizing principles of the human brain. Before you perform even the simplest movement, the pre-frontal cortex of your brain collaborates with a host of other brain structures to establish in neural space the goal of the movement. Goal setting is also psychologically important: Your journey, including your exercise program, remains aimless without a destination, and that destination is your goal.

Goals naturally vary with the individual. If looking good in a bikini is what gets you to the gym, excellent. If losing back, knee, or groin fat works for you, that's fine, too. If losing weight so you can fit into that stored wardrobe does the trick, great. As long as it motivates you and serves as a compass, it is a useful goal. And you don't have to tell another soul—just make your goals conscious to yourself. Take a few minutes now to list the major goals that would best motivate and guide your IBC program.

It is likely that the goals you list will either give you pleasure or avoid pain. Goals work to the extent that they provide reinforcement. In the carrot-and-stick metaphor, the carrot is reward, or positive reinforcement, while the stick is punishment, or negative reinforcement. Psychologists believe that reinforcement is the main engine of learned behavior, and that includes exercise adherence. To apply reinforcement in practice, figure out what is reward or punishment for you, and then build that into your exercise program in the form of specific goals.

Your next motivational tool is stimulus control. That means you consciously create sensory stimuli that support your IBC program. Some people pack their workout bag the night before, for example, and set it by the door. The early-morning stimulus of seeing the packed bag makes working out seem predestined, and it becomes difficult not to exercise. An exercise partner can be a persuasive stimulus control for some, as is reserving a special, inviolate time for exercise. You can implement stimulus control by writing notes to yourself, rewarding yourself when you reach specific milestones, changing your diet to include more things you like, and so on. As you learn what reinforcement works for you, you will also know what stimuli are most helpful in supporting your IBC program.

IBC incorporates stimulus control in several ways. When you prescribe the workload for your next workout during the current one, using the IBC method of progression, you create a stimulus that leaves no doubt about your path. Such stimulus control helps eliminate any possibility of indecision or wavering. Counting the circles that you draw around advances on your workout logs (chapter 6) is a form of stimulus control, as are the workout logs themselves. Take a few minutes now to make a list of stimuli that might help initiate and sustain your IBC program.

Contracting is the next tool in your motivation tool kit. Make a deal that supports your IBC program. The IBC method of progression, in which you prescribe your next workout and therefore make a contract with yourself, is an example. You can also make a contract with a workout partner, friend, personal trainer, child, or spouse. Any deal will do, as long as it has meaning to you and you can keep it. Start with modest terms, such as meeting the surgeon general's minimum exercise program, or working out two times a week for a month, or graduating from the beginning IBC level, or just completing the cardio phase. Later you can raise the bar by modifying and extending your contract (shaping).

Contracting is a subset of your next motivational tool, developing cognitive strategies. It sounds complex, but it again reduces to implementing the mind–body connection. Simply figure out a plan that supports your IBC program. Cognitive strategies can take many forms. For example, you can evaluate your reinforcements for physical activity, create a set of personalized exercise goals, apply the learn–heed–change process (figure 8.3) to exorcise demotivation demons, memorize or recite the Myth Busters—there are endless opportunities. The IBC Myth Busters are part of a cognitive strategy that helps create and maintain a constructive belief complex to support IBC workouts. Take the time now to develop and write down cognitive strategies that can support your IBC program.

Stick with It: Exercise Adherence

The key to a successful exercise program is adherence over the long term. Research has identified several factors that support exercise adherence, including enjoyment, efficiency, progression, variety, and freedom from pain and injury. It also helps to have a regular routine, good instruction, encouragement, group camaraderie, and social support. Let's identify these and see how IBC incorporates them.

First on the list of exercise adherence tools is social support. Our genes are those of a social animal, so it is not surprising that social support is such an important predictor of exercise initiation and adherence. A workout partner, group, or team, or a personal trainer—each provides a measure of social support that can assist exercise adherence. Even if you elect to work out alone, exercise adherence is almost twice as great when your partner approves. You can develop social support using a cognitive strategy. Discuss your exercise plans and program with the people you love—your significant other, friends, and family. Tell them how important your exercise program is to your well-being, and discuss how it can benefit them. Keep them apprised of how it is going and how it is changing your life. Such a cognitive strategy may even gain you a workout partner.

Second on the list of exercise adherence tools is self-management—meaning you become your own behavioral therapist. Figure out what makes you tick, and manage your behavior so that your exercise program becomes an integral part of your life. You are in a position to know yourself better than anyone, and you can best determine what will work to get you started with IBC and keep it going. You self-manage when you identify what you want, formulate it as a goal, and adopt behaviors to reach it. Self-management strategies include identifying effective reinforcements. These motivators of behavior tend to change over time, however. The quest for the body beautiful or athletic prowess in youth evolves in middle age toward sustaining capacities, and in old age toward maintaining mobility and maximizing independence. The unending flux of life challenges you to stay current with yourself. It takes work to create and sustain a constantly changing goal regime, but that is what will keep your IBC program active for life.

Peak Performance as a Motivation Tool

Peak performance milestones are an excellent motivational tool for anyone, at any level, from advanced exercisers and athletes (chapter 6) to deconditioned seniors (chapter 9). When you incorporate peak performance into your exercise program, you implement in one stroke several of the motivational and adherence strategies discussed above. For example, designing peak performance milestones for yourself is a cognitive strategy that requires and practices self-management. It also exemplifies goal setting, provides positive reinforcement, represents a form of stimulus control, corresponds to contracting with yourself, and can contribute to relapse prevention. As you reach your individual goals, you can identify new, higher peak performance milestones through shaping. Peak performance broadly engages the full gamut of motivation tools, which is why it can be useful at any exercise level.

To implement peak performance at any level of exercise, simply maximize any aspect of your performance at that level. You can integrate peak performance milestones into your IBC program from the beginning, or add them at any time. The definition of peak performance varies with genetics, age, and level, and individual performance milestones vary accordingly. If you are a deconditioned 70-year-old, peak performance may be as seemingly modest as reducing incontinence, increasing bone mineral density, or just living independently. If you are a beginning exerciser and your primary exercise goals are health and wellness, peak performance may consist of attaining above-average aerobic capacity for your age group. Simple tests to measure aerobic capacity, together with normative tables showing percentile rankings, are provided in the appendix to chapter 9. Your peak performance milestone then becomes a motivational tool, a challenge, a prod, a carrot that draws you ever closer to your overall exercise goal of health and wellness—and when you reach it, you can set the bar higher if you want (shaping).

At the level of the intermediate IBC program, a 30-year-old man of moderate genetic potential might set a peak performance milestone of completing a marathon. You can also establish peak performance milestones of surpassing a particular percentile ranking in strength and endurance measures for your age group. Normative tables showing percentile values are available for a great variety of exercises, including push-ups, abdominal curl-ups, and several resistance exercises with free weights or machines. These tables are posted at www.MiracleWorkout.com (click on "Performance") for your use in developing your personal peak performance milestones.

As you gain in aerobic power, strength, and endurance, and are able to move to the advanced level, peak performance milestones change, too. At advanced levels you are subject to the reality of diminishing returns, but there are countless peak performance options still available. A 25-year-old professional tennis player, for example, may set a milestone of a 100-mile-per-hour service. A 50-year-old woman with high genetic potential might define peak performance as achieving the 90th percentile level for physical strength and endurance for a younger age group.

Once you have achieved your advanced peak performance milestone, where do you go from there? That will depend on your circumstances, preferences, and imagination. I like trying to break old personal peak performance milestones, such as the one-repetition maximum levels that I set when I was younger, which gives me a feeling of accomplishment that is motivating. I also set a peak performance milestone of keeping up with the college athletes whom I train, both in individual exercises and in total workout workload. The friendly competition keeps me motivated and is a source of camaraderie. If you are an athlete, you can incorporate peak performance into the training for or achievement in your sport, or perhaps even excelling in a different sport. Your imagination is the only limit to finding peak performance milestones that will keep you interested and progressing at any level.

Relapse Prevention and Recovery

Life has a way of throwing curves that can disrupt even the best-intentioned and best-motivated exercise program. Relapses tend to occur at those transition points in life known as passages. There are enough of these to keep us busy for a lifetime. They include births and deaths, weddings and divorces, professional successes and failures, and even business trips or vacations. A crucial passage occurs, for example, upon graduation. First-year college students gain on the average 15 pounds—the so-called freshman 15—owing to the change in diet and exercise. If you are aware in advance that regular exercise will ensure more fun in college, promote better grades, provide more free time, and make your graduation more likely, you may be less likely to suffer a relapse at this critical juncture. Indeed, just becoming aware of the freshman 15 may be all the stimulus control and motivation you need.

Recognizing and planning for vulnerable passages is central to relapse prevention. Start before a relapse occurs—the preventive approach—by learning to identify those conditions that derail exercise programs and then creating a cognitive strategy to deal with them before they arise. In doing this, you can become your own behavioral therapist (self-management), or get help from a personal trainer. Nobody is perfect, however, so you will probably eventually suffer at least a partial relapse. You will then need the tools for recovering and getting back on track—or relapse recovery.

The key to successful relapse recovery is to treat a relapse not as a failure, but as an opportunity to learn something about yourself and a challenge to reestablish your exercise routine. When you stay focused on your long-term purpose, which is to prevent a relapse from becoming permanent, you convert the smallest step backward into resumption of your exercise program, your self-efficacy will increase, and you will be back on track stronger than ever.

Take a few moments now to list the relapse vulnerabilities that loom large for you, and develop strategies for dealing with them. One strategy might be to promise yourself never to drop below the surgeon general's minimum of 30 minutes of moderate exercise, three to five days per week, regardless of the challenges that life presents. You can fulfill this simple contract anywhere, any time—on vacation with your family, as an alternative way to get to work, or during job-related travel. A brisk walk is generally possible regardless of where you are, or what kind of pressures you face. It may even help put those pressures in better perspective.

Toward an Integrated Life

Evolution never intended for us to compartmentalize our exercise to three work-outs per week of 30 minutes each. Our genes expect and need more. Ultimately, we—and the culture we inhabit—need to revise our way of thinking (a cognitive strategy) and generalize our exercise behavior to as much of our life as possible. Start simply, by taking walks at sunset or before dinner. Trade the elevator for stairs whenever practicable. Park in the far corner of the parking lot, and walk rather than drive whenever possible. Get a bike, grow a garden, and choose a phys-ically active vacation in the mountains or high desert rather than a sedentary hol-iday by the side of a pool.

Professional pressure or lack of time need never derail your exercise program. Mikhail Gorbachev had perhaps the hardest job on earth—leading a massive and diverse nation while dismantling communism peacefully—yet he and his wife, Raisa, remained committed to a daily one-hour talk walk, in which they shared their day and discussed current issues and options. They combined exercise with relationship and profession, in an inspiring example of how to integrate regular exercise into a demanding professional schedule.

Take the time now to evaluate the pattern of your life in order to discover opportunities to generalize your exercise behavior. Nature intended us to integrate exercise into everyday life, and if you use your imagination, you will find dozens of ways to do that. It is a part of what we will develop shortly as the integrated approach to life.

9

Special Populations and Conditions

All people need exercise in this modern world, and all can reap rewards from IBC. The specifics of each exercise program differ, however, because people have different starting points, abilities, risks, limitations, and preferences. Certain groups also face unique circumstances, and if you belong to one of these, you may have special needs and require specific safety precautions. Even if you do not belong to such a special population, you may someday, and you no doubt know or love someone who does or will. This chapter will help you find the IBC workout that is right regardless of your unique circumstances.

Special Populations

The term *special populations* traditionally refers to groups who have particular clinical risks associated with health or body weight. Exercise professionals are increasingly casting the net wider, however, to include any identifiable group of people who benefit from or require special exercise procedures or precautions. This includes not only clinical cases but also children, the aged, and, increasingly, healthy women, particularly female athletes. According to a recent consensus statement of sports physicians,

> *Female athletes experience musculoskeletal injuries and medical problems, resulting from and/or impacting athletic activity. Team physicians must understand the gender-specific implications of these issues.*[1]

In this chapter, we will consider how to benefit from integrated exercise if you are a member of any special population. We'll also consider those environmental and circumstantial conditions—heat, humidity, and cold, for example—that any exerciser may encounter and should know how to handle. These conditions apply to everyone who exercises, whether or not you belong to a special population.

Reducing Risks of Exercise for Healthy Women

Regular exercise reduces risks to which women are particularly or uniquely subject, such as breast cancer, heart disease, and osteoporosis. Doctors recognize increasingly, however, that women are also subject to special conditions that create exercise risks. A recent consensus statement of team physicians representing the American College of Sports Medicine (ACSM) identified several such conditions or risks, including knee injuries, shoulder injuries, changes in the menstrual cycle, reproductive biology, eating disorders, risks associated with pregnancy, stress fractures, and osteoporosis. Here we'll examine the most important of these to learn how your IBC program can accommodate them.

Joint Injuries.

Female exercisers are more susceptible to knee injuries, including injuries to the anterior cruciate ligament (ACL) and patellofemoral joint of the knee. The ACL is a thick strand of connective tissue that originates on the femur and attaches to the tibia, and helps hold your knee together; the patellofemoral joint extends from the top to the bottom of the kneecap. The rate of noncontact ACL injuries in female athletes is 2–10 times higher than in their male counterparts. High-risk sports for knee injury in females athletes include soccer, basketball, skiing, lacrosse, and field hockey. Causes of elevated risk for knee injury in female athletes are multiple, including biomechanical—women have a lower center of gravity—and hormonal—including natural changes during the menstrual cycle, such as joints that are looser, or lax.

ACL injuries in women athletes "are amenable to prevention with specific conditioning programs."[2] One of the best approaches is to strengthen the knee with specific resistance exercises that target the ACL (for instance, figure 4.5, exercises 1–3). The leg extension exercise (figure 6.5, exercise 2) stresses the ACL, particularly at maximal extension, and therefore merits care when using heavy weights. Treadmill running for only 15 minutes increases joint laxity in women, which can increase the risk of the leg extension exercise. Joint laxity may vary during the menstrual cycle, particularly around the time of ovulation when blood estrogen peaks (see below). Leg extension is what strengthens the knee to reduce injury risk, but merits caution if you heat up or cardio-accelerate with treadmill running, if you have a history of knee injury, and around the time of ovulation.

Some older research seemed to indicate that weight-bearing exercises such as leg presses and squats, in which the knee is forced together by the load (called closed-chain kinetic exercises), were more effective and less risky than non-weight-bearing exercises such as leg extensions, which leave the knee joint uncompressed during muscle contraction (open-chain kinetic exercises). The preponderance of recent research, however, concludes that there is little or no difference in risk between closed- and open-chain exercise, and no difference in functional improvement during rehabilitation from knee surgery.

Women athletes are also at greater risk from shoulder injuries. The risk is greatest in sports such as volleyball, but occurs in swimming, tennis, and gymnastics as well. Women are more prone to shoulder injury owing to a combination of specific risk factors, including increased joint laxity, increased flexibility (range of motion), and decreased upper body strength. The solution is proper exercise, in this case specific shoulder workouts such as the bench press (figure 4.5, exercise 5), overhead or military press (figure 4.5, exercise 6), shoulder shrugs (figure 5.4, exercise 5), and deltoid exercises (figure 5.4, exercises 6–8). These exercises will strengthen shoulder muscles and tighten the joint, reducing the risk of injury.

The increased risk of leg and shoulder joint injury in women may result in part from natural hormonal changes associated with female reproductive biology, and particularly to the hormonal fluctuations during the menstrual cycle. Unfortunately, the exact cause, and even the effect, is less than clear. At least two studies have suggested that estrogen, which peaks around ovulation, is directly involved. Another study, however, reported increased risk of ACL injury during the luteal phase of the menstrual cycle, immediately prior to menstruation. Yet another study suggests no differences in strength or endurance associated with the menstrual cycle.

Pending further research to clarify these hormonally related risks, two characteristics of IBC ameliorate risks of joint injury in women. The first is body consciousness. The IBC method of progression draws attention to perceived pain and perceived exertion, bringing any early warning signs of knee or shoulder joint injury to your consciousness at the first hint of trouble. The second helpful feature of IBC for injury mitigation is the balance principle. Strengthening all the joints and muscles evenly is an ideal way to minimize the risks of joint injuries to which women are susceptible.

Reproductive Biology.

Women exercisers are also subject to risks associated with reproductive biology, including delayed onset of menstruation—sometimes past the age of 16 in female athletes at advanced levels. Intensive exercise can be associated also with other menstrual disruption, including cessation in absence of pregnancy and changes in the frequency or duration of periods. Cessation of menstruation for prolonged periods (three months or more) occurs in 2–5 percent of the general female population of reproductive age, but in up to 40 percent of women who participate in some sports. According to the consensus statement of the American College of Sports Medicine, menstrual dysfunction is at least two to three times more common in women athletes than in nonathletes, and 10–15 percent experience cessation or reduced frequency of periods.

The causes of these exercise-related impacts on the menstrual cycle are unknown, but body composition, and particularly the ratio of lean body mass to fat, may contribute. Sports that place a premium on low weight or appearance, such as distance running, ballet, bodybuilding, and gymnastics, have greater probabilities of altering or interrupting the menstrual cycle. According to the energy drain hypothesis, the menstrual cycle is disrupted when metabolic energy expended exceeds food energy consumed, resulting in loss of body fat. Increased caloric intake during intensive physical training may therefore help resolve this source of menstrual dysfunction.

Menstrual dysfunction can also signify low estrogen and/or progesterone levels, which reduce bone mineral density and can cause osteoporosis. It is not clear whether this is fully reversible following menopause—that is currently a matter of scientific debate and ongoing research. For this reason alone, early detection and treatment of menstrual dysfunction is important, whether or not it is associated with or caused by intense exercise. According to the ACSM, a comprehensive evaluation includes:

> *assessment for other causes of menstrual dysfunction, detailed menstrual, nutrition, and medication history; laboratory testing; and additional diagnostic testing as necessary.*[3]

Treatment options may include increased caloric intake, decreased energy expenditure, and hormone supplementation. Based on current scientific knowledge, body fat in the 17–22 percent range appears to contribute to normal menstrual function for athletes and nonathletic women alike.

Female athletes whose menstrual periods slow or stop are not necessarily at health risk. Some researchers believe that delayed onset of menstruation, as often occurs in young female athletes, could be a positive health benefit, because it is associated with reduced incidence of breast, cervical, and ovarian cancers later in life. Lower body fat in young female athletes supports less conversion of androgens to estrogen, and lower estrogen may result over a lifetime in a lower risk of the indicated cancers. Neither is cessation of periods necessarily a problem. Many mammalian species stop menstruating when food is scarce and body fat declines, ensuring that offspring are born only in times of proven abundance. An intense workout also releases a host of female hormones with anti-reproductive properties. As a general rule, however, if you are a heavy exerciser (intermediate or advanced IBC) and experience menstrual irregularities, see your doctor.

Eating Disorders.

Women who exercise intensely are at special risk for a linked combination of disordered eating behaviors termed the female athlete triad. This syndrome causes reduced body mass, abnormal or absent menstrual periods, and bone loss or osteoporosis. Disordered eating is a general risk among some women anyway, owing to unhelpful cultural stereotypes about body shape and size. The female athlete triad syndrome is a particular risk among women athletes who participate in sports that place a premium on low body weight, such as distance running, gymnastics, ballet, cheerleading, figure skating, and bodybuilding. In these sports, the prevalence of one or more components of the female athlete triad is 15–60 percent.

The first warning sign of eating disorders is an abnormal obsession that can eventually become pathological preoccupation with body weight and/or appearance. The obsession can progress to anorexia nervosa ("nervous loss of appetite"), bulimia nervosa ("ox hunger," or gorging followed by purging), or binge-eating disorder (gorging without subsequent purging). These eating disorders can disrupt the menstrual cycle and induce radical bone loss, increasing susceptibility to stress fractures and joint problems. Inadequate calcium intake exacerbates osteoporosis, and calcium supplementation and a commitment to normal food intake provide a partial solution. The recommended short-term solution to eating disorders is a combination of behavior modification, psychotherapy, and lowered physical activity levels. The long-term resolution to the female athlete triad is proper nutrition combined with exercise, particularly resistance training, and ongoing psychological support.

Osteoporosis.

Half of all women eventually develop osteoporosis. The female hormone estrogen enhances calcium absorption and limits its reabsorption from bone, so postmenopausal women who have reduced estrogen are at increased risk of osteoporosis. The benefits of exercise to female skeletal health are increasingly clear.

Moderate-to-high-intensity aerobic exercise . . . performed 3 days a week for 50 to 60 minutes each workout builds bone and retards its rate of loss.

Muscle-strengthening exercise also benefits bone mass. Individuals with greater back strength, and who train regularly with resistance exercise, have a greater spinal bone mineral content than weaker and untrained individuals.[4]

Although the benefits of exercise in general and weight training in particular for bone mineral density are abundant, too much of the same high-intensity training maintained over many years increases the risk of osteoporosis. As long as you do not exceed the intensity or frequency of the advanced IBC program described in chapter 6, and as long as you vary and periodize your IBC program as recommended and eat a complete diet, IBC should strengthen your bones and reduce the risk of osteoporosis for life.

Exercise During Pregnancy

Only your doctor can advise you competently regarding the health needs of you and your baby during pregnancy. Prenatal care is beyond the competence of your coach, personal trainer, or team physician. Exercise prescriptions change during pregnancy, however, and coaches, personal trainers, and female exercisers should all be aware of the changes recommended generally by exercise and health professionals. All research to date supports the view that "healthy women with uncomplicated pregnancy do not need to limit their exercise for fear of adverse effects."[5] Above all, the purpose and focus of exercise during pregnancy is to maintain or improve maternal fitness without endangering mother or child. Exercise prescriptions change as required to serve this goal.

Exercise during pregnancy, although modified, carries profound benefits to both mother and child. The American College of Obstetricians and Gynecologists recommends regular exercise during pregnancy at least three times a week. In one study on nearly 10,000 pregnant women, 42 percent reported that they exercised regularly, a substantially greater percentage than among the general population. Exercise throughout pregnancy can help sustain aerobic and muscle fitness, control weight, decrease back pain, improve energy levels and sleep patterns, strengthen childbirth muscles, reduce the number of doctor visits and interventions, shorten labor and make it less painful, and facilitate recovery following childbirth. Exercise is good for your baby, too. Children born of mothers who exercise have on average lower body fat and score higher on standard intelligence tests.

Exercise during pregnancy also carries risks, however. These include potential uterine trauma, dehydration, environmental exposure, and hypoxia (reduced oxygen availability). In addition, exercise interacts with normal physiological changes during pregnancy, including weight gain, musculoskeletal changes, and altered cardiovascular physiology, including increased heart rate and increased oxygen demand. Exercise during pregnancy therefore requires knowledgeable monitoring.

To mitigate risks, follow these four steps: First, as soon as you find out you are pregnant, consult with your personal physician about the exercise program that is appropriate for you. Second, do not exercise in the supine position (lying on your back) after the first trimester (12th–14th weeks) of pregnancy. Exercise in the supine position during pregnancy can interfere with the circulation of blood and oxygen to you and your baby. Third, if you exercise at vigorous levels, ask your doctor whether you should reduce its intensity to moderate to ensure adequate uterine blood and oxygen flow. Fourth, with your doctor's guidance, make sure your diet is adequate to the double demands of exercise and pregnancy—especially calories, iron, calcium, and folic acid. You need 300 Kcal per day beyond your normal caloric intake to support your growing child. Insufficient weight gain—less than 1 kilogram (2.2 pounds) per month during the last two trimesters—may signify an imbalance in nutrition and exercise.

A longer, moderate IBC workout during pregnancy can be as beneficial to mother and child as a shorter vigorous workout, may carry fewer risks to both, and can achieve an adequate training effect. Do not attempt to progress at the maximum rate during pregnancy—there will be plenty of time for that later—and, instead, shift toward maintenance mode. Be attentive to any signs of trouble— bloody or fluid vaginal discharge, swelling of extremities, unilateral pain, abdominal pain or premature contractions, abnormal heart rate—and seek medical advice if any occur. IBC's use of biofeedback (Rating of Perceived Pain, Rating of Perceived Exertion, heart rate) is just what you need to help detect warning signs during pregnancy. After your baby is born, you can generally resume your normal workout gradually, starting four to six weeks postpartum, if your doctor agrees. That is the fastest way back to your usual strength, endurance, and body composition, and it may help you beat the baby blues—postpartum depression that afflicts 80 percent of new mothers.

The Overweight and Obese

You can determine whether you fit the clinical description for obesity by calculating your Body Mass Index (BMI) using the procedure in the appendix to chapter 5, or the online calculator at www.MiracleWorkout.com (click on "BMI Calculator"). People who are overweight (BMI greater than 25 but less than 30) need take no special precautions during exercise beyond those detailed in chapters 4–6. If you are clinically obese, however (BMI greater than 30), you may benefit even more from IBC. According to the American College of Sports Medicine,

A continued physical activity program appears to be the best predictor of long-term weight-loss and its subsequent maintenance.[6]

The first step to addressing obesity is to understand its causes. Everyone, not just the obese, should be aware that gluttony is not the usual cause of obesity. According to one source, Americans consume 5–10 percent fewer calories now than in 1980, yet average body weight over the same period increased by 2–4 kilograms (5–10 pounds). Several studies on adults and children alike suggest that obese and nonobese people typically eat the same amount; the main difference between them is in the level of physical activity.

Genetic and cultural influences may account for up to 50 percent of obesity. People who are obese often have a blunted thermic response to a meal—their metabolism does not increase as much as that of a nonobese person after eating—which can account for a weight gain of many pounds per year over a lifetime. Sedentary lifestyle and/or bad experiences with exercise account for most other cases of obesity. Television is a primary contributor—every hour per week of watching television raises the prevalence of obesity by 2 percent, and the average child spends up to 26 hours per week watching TV, about the same time spent in school. Reversing obesity requires more exercise, less TV, and a healthy diet.

Obese people tend to be exercise averse, however, creating a chicken-and-egg conundrum. The reasons for exercise avoidance by the obese range from low self-esteem to bad past experiences with exercise. There is also a practical consideration—it is harder to exercise when you are obese. At any given exercise workload, the heart has to pump harder, blood pressure is higher, and the lungs have to work harder during even moderate exercise. Obesity is often associated with restricted lung volume, which can create difficulty breathing during intense or aerobic exercise. Any given work task, including exercise, therefore feels harder, which can be disheartening.

Obesity typically begins in childhood, and an obese child typically becomes an obese adult. Weight loss programs seldom have the desired long-term effects for obese people. You can successfully break the mold, but the best and indeed only solution for children and adults alike is a long-term change in lifestyle that prioritizes regular exercise. Limit yourself to low-impact workouts at first. High-impact exercises create sudden bone or joint stress, and extra body weight increases susceptibility to bone or joint injury. Stationary cycles and elliptical trainers are preferable to jogging or running. Be attentive also to environmental considerations such as heat and humidity (see Special Environmental Considerations, below), because adipose tissue is a good insulator, and too much can interfere with heat regulation during exercise.

Above all, combat obesity by committing for the long haul. Reversing obesity implies that you are recovering from a lifetime of relative inactivity and a mind-set that accompanies a sedentary lifestyle. Obesity typically takes a lifetime to develop. Therefore it takes a lifetime commitment to physical activity and proper diet to reverse. A good starting point is daily walking for a few weeks or months, followed when you're ready by the moderate exercise of the beginning IBC program.

Combine this moderate exercise with good dietary practices (chapter 10). Every 3,500 calories that you consume below your normal expenditure will shed 1 pound, and that means you'll shed 1 pound every week that you shave 500 Kcal from your normal daily equilibrium diet. Starvation diets are counterproductive (chapter 2). Nutrition experts recommend that you never consume fewer than 1,200 Kcal a day, and never attempt to shed more than 2 pounds a week, 1,000 calories below your daily equilibrium diet. If you consume 500 calories less than you burn each day, you can, in principle, lose 50 pounds a year. That will make it easier to graduate to the more vigorous exercise of the intermediate IBC program, and you can be on your way to overcoming obesity.

The Young

Exercise in youth is crucial, because lifetime patterns of physical activity or inactivity form during childhood. Adult obesity, for example, usually starts in childhood with sedentary lifestyles and unhealthy dietary practices. The very act of expending physical energy as a child, in combination with appropriate eating habits, is the antidote to adult obesity. In addition, crucial developmental events that require exercise take place during childhood. For example, fully a quarter of Bone Mineral Deposition (BMD) occurs during just two years of childhood, and exercise is one of the best stimuli. On this basis, exercise physiologists have suggested that the cure for osteoporosis is properly the province of childhood (pediatric medicine) rather than old age (geriatric medicine).

The National Association for Sport and Physical Education recommends that elementary school children accumulate at least 60 minutes, and up to several hours, of exercise every day, including intermittent 10–15 minute bursts of moderate to vigorous exercise alternating with rest and recovery. We are far from meeting these recommendations, however. A recent study of elementary school children in California found that only 25 percent achieved age-appropriate standards for aerobic capacity in 1-mile walk and run tests.

Physical education in schools is deprioritized, unfortunately, and for all the wrong reasons. A focus on academic achievement is displacing physical education, in the mistaken belief that scholastic performance is unrelated to physical fitness. It's not—the mind–body connection works during childhood, too, and children who get enough exercise may also show better academic performance. Tight budgets all too readily displace physical education instruction, when in fact the costs to society of inadequate physical activity during childhood are staggering and threaten to overwhelm medical systems and government budgets (chapter 10).

When it comes to exercise in children, and its guidance by grown-ups, "children are not small adults."[7] There are special precautions to follow. In comparison with adults, children

- Have limited anaerobic capacities owing to biochemical differences.
- Have immature cardiopulmonary systems—their lungs are less developed and less efficient.
- Use more energy (and therefore generate more heat) and fatigue more easily during typical aerobic tasks such as walking or running.
- Have immature cardiovascular systems and therefore dissipate heat less effectively than adults.
- Don't sweat as much, owing to a less developed sweat response, decreasing their capacity to acclimatize to heat.
- Mistakenly perceive that they acclimatize to heat faster than they can, increasing the risk of heat-related ailments.
- Are more subject to overuse injuries owing to ongoing growth, particularly of bones and muscles.
- Have limited attention spans and less tolerance for activity that is not enjoyable.

The guiding goal of exercise for children is to foster love of movement and physical activity, and to develop healthy, lifelong exercise habits. Effective exercise programs for children must take into account the above special characteristics. Aside from enjoyment, the most salient precaution in view of the above physiological differences is to ensure adequate hydration and limited exercise (or frequent breaks) during hot or humid weather. Healthy children of normal weight generally do not need a heart rate prescription, nor do they require cardiovascular risk stratification (chapter 5), because they are generally in the low-risk category and naturally adjust the intensity of their exercise to their own capacities.

Above all, encourage kids to play in natural activities as much as possible. When left to their own devices, kids tend to self-regulate effectively. They will set their own tempo, if the opportunities are available and if sedentary alternatives such as television are discouraged. Girls may still need greater support for physical activity to counter lingering cultural stereotypes. Children generally prefer group activities over individual exercise pursuits, and they should participate in programs that prepare them with appropriate motor and sport skills to last a life-time.

Specific activity recommendations for children include aerobic exercise at 50–80 percent of maximum functional capacity for 30–60 minutes three to five days a week. Natural play activities suffice, but resistance training is increasingly popular among older children, in large part because they like looking buff. Unfortunately, performance-enhancing drugs such as steroids are increasingly available and accessible to children. Resistance training for children should therefore include a thorough education in the hazards and follies of drugs (chapter 10).

The recommended guidelines for resistance training in children differ with age. Between the years of 5 and 10, it is recommended that kids focus on the elements of form, with an emphasis on supervised multijoint or natural movements rather than isolation machines, light weights, and many repetitions. Between the ages of 10 and 16 children weightlifters can grow into more advanced exercise, add sport-specific components, and increase volume. If children do resistance training, they should balance it with aerobic exercise. Young adults are ready for systematic programs such as beginning IBC. By the age of 16, adult-style programs like the intermediate or advanced IBC programs become more appropriate.

The Elderly

You can definitely be too young for IBC, but you can never be too old. Seniors can remain active and do even the advanced IBC program well into old age. Some authorities classify seniors as a special population, but treating elders differently for purposes of exercise may be a cultural habit and not a biological necessity. Aside from the initial health screening procedures and risk stratification process (chapters 4–5), there is little or no need for any different prescriptions for elders unless physical capacities are already limited or other special medical conditions apply.

In one of many published studies on weightlifting seniors, people whose average age was 90.2 years showed a 170 percent gain in strength over an 8-week training period, more than 20 percent per week—a doubling time of less than a month. Strength gains in these seniors showed no tendency to plateau during training, and were similar for men and women. Another research study focused on 100 frail nursing home residents whose average age was 87. Their muscular strength doubled in only 10 weeks of resistance training for 45 minutes, 3 times a week. Strength training is clearly effective even for the most aged and frail exerciser. As long as health is not an issue, there is no physiological reason why seniors cannot work up to the advanced IBC program.

Deconditioned seniors recovering from a lifetime of inactivity should start slowly and advance gradually to moderate and finally to brisk walking. When you reach the point that you can walk at a brisk pace for 30 continuous minutes, you are ready for the beginning IBC program (chapter 4). Many seniors prefer group exercise programs—the social interaction can be as important as the physical activity—and IBC lends itself perfectly to group workouts. Our swim coach at the University of California, Kim Musch, devised an efficient group IBC program that could work great for any group, including seniors. He matches his swimmers in pairs, who then alternate a specific cardio machine and resistance exercise during IBC. If cardio machines are limiting, marching in place or other inexpensive, nonmotorized options can be alternated with simple resistance exercises using dumbbells and body weight, as well as ROM exercise, for an entertaining and healthy senior workout group.

Water-based exercise can be ideal for deconditioned seniors because there is less impact on joints. You can alternate stationary kicking or running in place in water (water sprinting) for cardio-acceleration with water ROM or other pool-based exercises. With minimum guidance from trained personnel, a group of seniors could learn and apply the principles of IBC and then devise their own group programs to incorporate them. The process exercises both the mind and the body, and the only limit is the imagination!

Safety considerations for exercise in seniors are similar to those for younger adults, as outlined in chapter 4–6 and their appendices. The primary exception is that older exercisers—men over 45 and women over 55—fall into the moderate cardiovascular risk category, leading to the recommendation by the American College of Sports Medicine that they obtain a doctor-supervised exam and medical test prior to vigorous exercise (chapter 5). Deconditioned seniors should start lower and build up more slowly than younger exercisers, particularly during resistance training, because aging joints, tendons, and ligaments are weak links. Deconditioned people can also expect the fastest gains, however, because they have so much room to improve.

Seniors are capable of all of the forms of exercise that younger adults do, and can achieve a high degree of aerobic fitness, strength, and muscle endurance. According to the American College of Sports Medicine, "while aging is inevitable, both the pace and potential reversibility of this process may be amenable to intervention."[8] In other words, you cannot stop aging, but you can slow it dramatically, and it is never too late to start. Instead of a long, steep decline in physical capabilities, you can sustain them to the end by rectangularizing the aging process.

Heavy exercise does not itself wear out joints that cause arthritis in aging people and older athletes. Chronic or repetitive high-impact exercise such as running can damage articular cartilage that separates abutting bones, as in the knees, leading to osteoarthritis. On the other hand, inactivity is equally or more damaging. Those cartilage-producing cells, the chondrocytes, need stimulation to maintain strong and healthy joints. Research suggests that athletes who develop osteoarthritis in later life do so not because of accumulated physical activity, but rather as a biological response to undiagnosed joint injuries.

> *The available evidence shows that moderate habitual exercise does not increase the risk of developing osteoarthritis, and carefully selected sports and exercise programs improve mobility and strength in older people and people with mild and moderate osteoarthritis.*[9]

Special Medical Populations

According to the American College of Sports Medicine, exercise is appropriate even for people with serious medical conditions, such as hypertension, peripheral vascular disease, pulmonary disease, diabetes, asthma, and various cardiac diseases. Exercise can even help Chronic Fatigue Syndrome (see the sidebar). Exercise prescription for special medical populations may include aerobic exercise, resistance training, and Range of Motion (ROM) exercises. If you belong to a special medical population, or if you are rehabilitating from illness or long inactivity, work with your doctor or physical therapist to ensure that any exercise you undertake is safe and appropriate for you.

Special Environmental Conditions

Environmental conditions—temperature, humidity, altitude, and pollution—can affect exercise performance and safety for all exercisers, but they are particularly important for vulnerable members of special populations. Cold stress or ambient pollution, for example, can trigger exercise-induced asthma in people with heightened bronchial reactivity. Children are particularly vulnerable owing to their relatively immature thermoregulatory systems. It is helpful for every exerciser to know the basics of special environmental conditions that affect exercise, and how best to cope with them.

Heat.

Heat stress is the greatest risk for most exercisers. The human body can tolerate an increase in temperature of only about 5 degrees Celsius (9 degrees Fahrenheit), and vigorous exercise raises core temperature by about 2 degrees C (nearly 4 degrees F). The safety margin is a slim 3 degrees C (5 degrees F). Exercise creates a biological competition between the body's heat regulatory mechanisms, which send blood to the surface to release heat, and exercise, which shunts blood to internal working muscles to feed and cleanse them. Each degree of increase in temper-

Myth Buster 9: Exercise and Illness

THE MYTH: Exercise is only for people who are already healthy and well.

If you belong to one of the "special populations" defined in this chapter, and particularly if you are a member of a clinically defined population or have a chronic illness, see your doctor before you start to exercise. Most people who can move, however, including those with chronic illnesses, are candidates for IBC and can benefit from doing it.

Consider, for example, one of the most mysterious and debilitating chronic illnesses, Chronic Fatigue Syndrome (CFS). It afflicts about 1 percent of the U.S. population—nearly three million people, mostly women. Although the cause is unknown, the main symptom is fatigue—unexplained, persistent, debilitating fatigue. Clinical diagnosis includes four or more of eight additional symptoms—short-term memory impairment, sore throat, tender cervical or axillary lymph nodes, muscle pain, multijoint pain without visible signs, headaches, unrefreshing sleep, and post-exertional malaise lasting 24 hours or more.

The current literature on Chronic Fatigue suggests only two effective interventions—cognitive behavioral therapy and exercise. If you suffer from CFS, or any other chronic illness, you may understandably find it harder to get started with exercise in the first place. It is not surprising that researchers find that CFS patients are either the same or less fit than control patients without CFS, because many CFS patients deliberately reduce their physical activity to avoid fatigue—just the opposite of what's needed to restore energy.

An approach recommended as effective by physicians includes moderate exercise guided by one of the same tools used in IBC—your Rating of Perceived Exertion (RPE). Because your symptoms may fluctuate from day to day, CFS sufferers are advised to adjust the intensity of exercise according to how hard it feels—RPE—and dispense with rigid goals and timetables. And take heart: In one study, CFS patients showed a 13 percent increase in aerobic capacity over a 4–6 month period. They reported less fatigue, increased functional capacity, a lower heart rate, and fewer symptoms. Doctors conclude that "Exercise appears to be a useful and effective form of therapy for patients with CFS."[10]

THE REALITY: Even people with debilitating chronic illnesses such as CFS may be able to benefit from IBC, under medical supervision.

The IBC Myth Buster

MYTH: Exercise is exclusively for the healthy and well.

FACT: IBC may be helpful for the infirm, but only with doctor approval and supervision.

ature above 24 degrees C (75 degrees F) raises heart rate about one Beat per Minute (BPM), potentially changing heart rate training windows. The American College of Sports Medicine recommends decreasing exercise dosage at temperatures above 27 degrees C (81 degrees F).

Heat stress has made headlines frequently in the past few years when professional athletes succumbed to it. In the past two decades, more than 100 football players have died from heat illnesses, although football uniforms and equipment are partly to blame because they reduce normal heat transfer by 50 percent. Heat has a special impact when humidity is high, because the moisture in the air works against the body's main regulatory response to heat—evaporative cooling through perspiration. The combination of high heat and temperature in tropical or semitropical environments can compromise outdoor exercise, including outdoor IBC workouts (chapter 7), and encourages workouts during the cooler morning or evening hours or in regulated indoor environments.

Heat illnesses range from heat cramps and fainting to heat exhaustion and heatstroke. Heat exhaustion has symptoms of unusual fatigue, flushed skin, profuse sweating, and abnormally high pulse rate. The appropriate first aid includes rest, cooling, and drink. Heatstroke is an acute medical emergency that entails lack of sweating, and even chills, and neurological deficits such as disorientation, seizures, and coma. The first aid includes aggressive cooling, rest, and immediate transport to a hospital for medical assistance. You can help mitigate or avoid these environmental hazards of exercise by proper hydration, applying body consciousness, following the recommendations of the ACSM—including postponing competitive endurance activities at ambient temperatures above 27 degrees C (81 degrees F)—and taking the necessary special precautions for special populations.

Cold.

Exercising in the cold is less a problem, because exercise itself creates internal heat that can sustain core temperature down to an ambient temperature of minus 30 degrees C (minus 22 degrees F) without heavy clothing. On the other hand, human thermoregulatory mechanisms protect primarily against heat, rather than cold, and humans adapt more successfully to chronic heat exposure than to regular cold. Breathing air below freezing can cause bronchial constriction in individuals with reactive air passages, leading to an asthma episode. Perhaps the most common general problem with cold-weather exercise is dehydration. Cold air holds less water, and so you lose more fluid breathing in a cold, dry environment. Cold also increases urine production and loss of fluid. The solution is to drink more water than usual. Hypothermia and frostbite can occur at temperatures below minus 30 degrees C, and outdoor exercise is not recommended under such extreme conditions.

Altitude.

Altitude is relevant to many exercisers, including skiers, mountain bikers, and backpackers. The main challenge of exercising at a higher altitude is that there is less oxygen, making the heart and lungs work harder at any given exercise intensity. The additional strain of exercise can be dangerous for people who already belong to a special population, particularly cardiac and pulmonary patients. Even for healthy people, a reduction of aerobic power at a high altitude reduces work capacity and endurance. Acclimatization helps—most healthy people get used to the lowered oxygen in a few days, although exercise is still harder than at sea level, as reflected by a feeling of breathlessness at high altitude and lower exercise capacity.

High-altitude illnesses include Acute Mountain Sickness (AMS) and the more serious High-Altitude Pulmonary Edema (HAPE) and High-Altitude Cerebral Edema (HACE). AMS symptoms include headache, nausea, and insomnia, and usually arise in susceptible people quickly, 6–12 hours after ascent to altitudes of 3,048 meters (10,000 feet) or higher. AMS usually abates after 3 to 7 days of acclimatization to altitude. HAPE is more serious and even life threatening, and exercise exacerbates the condition. It strikes about 2 percent of people who ascend to altitudes of 10,000 feet. Symptoms include a dry, raspy coughing and wheezing, followed by fluid retention. The required first aid is to descend immediately to lower altitude. HACE occurs in 1 percent of people who ascend above 2,700 meters (9,000 feet), includes exaggerated symptoms of AMS, and requires immediate descent.

Air Pollution.

Unclean air can be a challenge for outdoor exercisers in urban areas, where most people in industrialized countries now live. The only practical way to protect from the adverse impacts of air pollution during exercise is avoidance, which requires knowledge of daily and seasonal fluctuations in pollution. Radio stations in some urban areas report the Pollution Standards Index (PSI) or other indices of air quality. A PSI level above 100 is "unhealthful" for the general population. At that pollution level, members of special medical populations—and particularly people who suffer heart or lung ailments—should reduce outdoor activity, while members of the general population should avoid vigorous outdoor exercise. Indoor pollution, however, can also be problematic, particularly in humid environments, which encourage the growth of mold. If you live in such an area, make sure your health club or spa is free of internal condensation and visible signs of mold, and has adequate ventilation and filtering.

Peak Performance in Special Populations

Peak performance is the guiding goal of the advanced IBC program (chapter 6), but you do not have to cede this key motivational technique to the advanced exerciser or professional athlete. You can incorporate peak performance milestones into the most basic IBC program, whether you are a beginning exerciser, a member of a special population, or a deconditioned senior. For example, set for yourself a peak performance milestone of increasing your aerobic capacity to a new personal record. Recall from chapter 2 that aerobic power (VO_{2MAX}) is the maximum amount of oxygen your body can absorb and use during exercise. If your aerobic power is currently in the 10th percentile for your age group, for example, aim for the 50th percentile. If you are already there, go after the 90th percentile!

Start by measuring your aerobic capacity using the simple field test shown in the appendix to this chapter. All it takes is a measured 1-mile flat course, such as a high school track, and a stopwatch, followed by a simple calculation that will take just a few minutes. Complete the process by determining your current percentile ranking from the normative table of aerobic power, also shown in the appendix. That will tell you where you stand among the people in your age group and gender. After you have found your VO_{2MAX} and your percentile ranking, use it to set a peak performance milestone for yourself. If you are already at the 50th percentile for your age group, a reasonable (if ambitious) peak performance goal is to reach the 90th percentile.

You can set peak performance milestones using normative tables (population percentiles) or standards (excellent, good, and so on) for aerobic power as above, or for push-ups, curl-ups, and most basic resistance exercises. These tables are posted at www.MiracleWorkout.com, under "Performance." As you grow stronger, your level will increase, inviting you to raise the bar ever higher, and if you keep at this peak performance process for life, you can maximize your physical capacity well into old age.

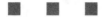

Appendix to Chapter 9

Measuring Your Aerobic Power*

The easiest field test for measuring your VO_{2MAX} is the one-mile Rockport Walking Test, which you can do if you can walk a mile comfortably. All you need is a measured one-mile course (four times around a conventional running track), a watch or stopwatch, your body weight, and fifteen or twenty minutes. Here is your simple three-step guide:

- **Walk** as fast as you can for one level mile, without jogging or running, and time yourself. Walking means your heel strikes the ground first at the end of the swing phase of each step. Most oval running tracks are 0.25 miles around, so four laps make a mile.
- **Count** your number of heartbeats during the last part of your walk or at the end of your walk for 15 seconds, using the radial pulse (wrist) method (chapter 4). Remember to start counting at zero, not one, to encompass the full 15-second period.
- **Calculate** your aerobic power by plugging your number of heartbeats into the equation below, along with the other variables indicated.

Equation: VO_{2MAX} (mL O_2 per kg per minute) = 132.853 − [0.1692 × (your body mass in pounds / 2.2)] − (0.3877 × your age) + (6.315 × 0 for females or × 1 for males) − (3.2649 × your time in minutes) − (0.1565 × the number of heartbeats you recorded in 15 seconds × 4). Do the calculations in brackets and parentheses first, as shown in the sample calculations below.

Sample Calculations of Aerobic Power (VO_{2MAX})

Women. Valerie is 62 years of age and weighs 155 lbs. She walked one mile as fast as she could in 15 minutes and 30 seconds. The number of heartbeats she counted in the final 15 seconds was 33. Her aerobic power is:

$$VO_{2MAX} = 132.853 - [0.1692 \times (155 \text{ lbs}/2.2 \text{ lbs/kg})] - (0.3877 \times 62) +$$
$$(6.315 \times 0) - (3.2649 \times 15.50 \text{ minutes}) - (0.1565 \times 33 \times 4)$$

---

* Adapted from G. M. Kline, J. P. Porcari, R. Hintermeister, et al. (1987). "Estimation of VO_{2MAX} from a one-mile track walk, gender, age, and body weight." *Med Sci Sports Exerc* 19, 253–259, cited from American College of Sports Medicine, *ACSM's Guidelines for Exercise Testing and Prescription,* sixth edition (Philadelphia: Lippincott Williams & Wilkins, 2000), table D-2, p. 307. Copyright © 2000 by American College of Sports Medicine. Reproduced by permission of Lippincott Williams & Wilkins.

TABLE 9.1
NORMATIVE TABLE FOR MAXIMUM AEROBIC POWER (VO$_{2MAX}$) BY AGE AND GENDER

Normative table for percentile values of maximal aerobic power (VO$_{2MAX}$ in units of mL O$_2$ per kg body weight per minute) for predominantly white, college-educated people of different ages.

	Age Group				
Percentile	20–29	30–39	40–49	50–59	60+
Men					
90	51.4	50.4	48.2	45.3	42.5
80	48.2	46.8	44.1	41.0	38.1
70	46.8	44.6	41.8	38.5	35.3
60	44.2	42.4	39.9	36.7	33.6
50	42.5	41.0	38.1	35.2	31.8
40	41.0	38.9	36.7	33.8	30.2
30	39.5	37.4	35.1	32.3	28.7
20	37.1	35.4	33.0	30.2	26.5
10	34.5	32.5	30.9	28.0	23.1
Women					
90	44.2	41.0	39.5	35.2	35.2
80	41.0	38.6	36.3	32.3	31.2
70	38.1	36.7	33.8	30.9	29.4
60	36.7	34.6	32.3	29.4	27.2
50	35.2	33.8	30.9	28.2	25.8
40	33.8	32.3	29.5	26.9	24.5
30	32.3	30.5	28.3	25.5	23.8
20	30.6	28.7	26.5	24.3	22.8
10	28.4	26.5	25.1	22.3	20.8

From American College of Sports Medicine, *ACSM's Guidelines for Exercise Testing and Prescription,* sixth edition (Philadelphia: Lippincott Williams & Wilkins, 2000), table 4-5, p. 77. Copyright © 2000 by American College of Sports Medicine. Reproduced by permission of Lippincott Williams & Wilkins.

$$= 132.853 - 11.921 - 24.037 + 0 - 50.606 - 20.658$$

$$= 25.631 \text{ mL O}_2 \text{ per kg body weight per minute}$$

Valerie's VO_{2MAX} value of 25.6 places her near the 50th percentile in aerobic power for her age group and gender (see the table). In other words, her aerobic power is equal to about half of all women in her age group.

Men. Harold is 72 years of age and weighs 160 lbs. He walked one mile as fast as he could in 17 minutes and 30 seconds. His number of heartbeats for the final fifteen seconds was 30. His aerobic power is:

$$VO_{2MAX} = 132.853 - [0.1692 \times (160 \text{ lbs})/(2.2 \text{ lbs/kg})] - (0.3877 \times 72) +$$
$$(6.315 \times 1) - (3.2649 \times 16.50 \text{ minutes}) - [0.1565 \times (30) \times (4)]$$

$$= 132.853 - 12.305 - 27.914 + 6.315 - 53.871 - 18.780$$

$$= 26.298 \text{ mL O}_2 \text{ per kg body weight per minute}$$

His VO_{2MAX} value of 26.298 places Harold near the twentieth percentile in aerobic power for his age group and gender (table). In other words, his aerobic power is greater than about one-fifth of all men in his age group.

10

The Integrated Life

Everything is connected to everything else, as we saw way back in chapter 2. This means that IBC will work miracles best when you adopt a systems approach to your whole life. All aspects of life are interrelated, and what's good for the whole is best for the parts. This chapter examines that broader context for IBC. Because everything is interconnected, the Miracle Workout does not work its miracles in a vacuum; what's required is an integrated life that addresses the full web that makes your life what it is, from diet and sleep to social institutions.

The Systems Approach to Life

The system that is each of us has at least four dimensions: physical, mental, emotional, and spiritual, all of which interact reciprocally, as surely as the parts of the human body interact with one another in mutual interdependence. To reach physical goals, we can no more ignore the mental, emotional, and spiritual dimensions than the muscles can ignore the heart or the brain or the lungs. All four dimensions of the human being interact seamlessly in the interconnected being that is each of us.

You already know about the mind–body connection. If you have already started your IBC program, you have also experienced its impact on the emotional body. You relate better to other people, sleep better, and wake up the next morning in a better mood. As with all interactions in any system, the exchanges are a two-way street. The physical supports the emotional, which benefits the physical. When you feel satisfied, you are more at peace with the world, you grow in self-efficacy, and you are more highly motivated to optimize your physical being—which feeds your self-efficacy in a constructive cycle of mutual reinforcement.

The spiritual dimension of the human being is integrated equally into this mutually dependent nexus. Eckhart Tolle writes that "all evils are the effect of unconsciousness."[1] One path to consciousness is to direct attention away from thinking and into the body or—as Tolle terms it—"Inhabiting the Body." He suggests that as long as we exist on the physical plane, spiritual transformation can take place only through the body and, in particular, its focus on the present moment.

The art of inner-body awareness will develop into a completely new way of living, a state of permanent connectedness with Being, and will add a depth to your life that you have never known before.[2]

The cultivation of body consciousness through IBC is one way to harness what Tolle terms "the Power of Now," directing attention inward and beyond.

The importance of body consciousness or awareness as a tool for spiritual development lies at the heart of Eastern traditions like Yoga, and the martial arts such as Aikido.

Conscious embodiment assists us in being present with the many experiences of our journey through life. Being more present in our bodies also allows our spirit to more fully inhabit our being. As we come more fully into our bodies, we are able to know and manifest our true purpose in life.[3]

Two thousand years ago a well-known Christian prophet portrayed the human body as the "temple of the spirit." If we accept this premise, either from religious conviction or personal persuasion, then we assume the responsibility to develop the gift of the body to the degree that we receive. IBC, and its practice of body consciousness, is one way to focus attention on the inner self, the now, and heighten personal consciousness.

Systems thinking extends beyond the four dimensions of the individual to the broader society, where we interact with the myriad customs, institutions, and people that make up the system of civilization. Social institutions such as schools, churches, hospitals, transportation, and the workplace all fit together in a continuous web of which we are part, and contribute to our relationship with our physical selves. The evidence mounts daily that unless we attend effectively to the physical dimension of self, society, and the planet as a whole, trying times lie ahead.

The Food Fight

The relation between diet and exercise exemplifies this interconnectedness. Inattention to one detracts from the other. This point emerges dramatically in Morgan Spurlock's film documentary *Super Size Me.* For one month, he ate nothing but McDonald's fast food to see what would happen to his body, and filmed the experience. He started the self-experiment in "supreme physical condition,"[4] but after three weeks on the all-McDonald's diet, his liver began to fail and his doctors advised him to end the experiment. He persevered, and within four weeks gained 25 pounds, saw his total cholesterol increase from 168 to 230, became depressed and listless, and felt

> *horrible—physically, psychologically and emotionally. I was ashen, pale, my energy level was low. Then I'd eat the food, I'd feel great, and an hour later I'd feel hungry again.*"[5]

Spurlock acknowledged that his experience was extreme, but also estimated that some people eat at McDonald's "three or four times a week." He's right on target—a study published in the January 2004 issue of *Pediatrics* by researchers at Harvard Medical School and the U.S. Department of Agriculture evaluated the diets of 6,212 U.S. children and adolescents. They discovered that on the average, they ate fast food two or three times a week. These and other studies paint a picture of a society at risk from not only how much we eat, but also what we eat.

The average American is understandably confused about diet. In fact, it has degenerated into a confusing debate in which successive generations are bombarded by contrasting diet claims, each portraying itself as the ultimate solution. As Dr. Dean Edell observes in his book *Life, Liberty, and the Pursuit of Healthiness,* there are only two kinds of diets: a low-carbohydrate, and therefore high-protein and -fat diet, or a high-carbohydrate, and therefore low-protein and -fat diet. The American public has been "driven crazy," in his words, by the fervent advocacy of one and then the other, by one set of authorities after another, for decades.

The Hunter-Gatherer Diet

Perhaps we can seek guidance from the same source we consulted for IBC, our hunter-gatherer ancestors, for exactly the same reason—we have their genes. In diet as in exercise, the evolutionary roots lie in the experience of our ancestors, encoded now in the genes they bequeathed us. The wide array of hunter-gatherer societies throughout human history furnishes nuggets of dietary wisdom. Thousands of independent hunter-gatherer bands, from the Abenakis to the Zaparos, colonized every conceivable environment, ecosystem, and corner of the earth. Remarkably, these primitive peoples were healthier than their brethren who first turned to farming.

> *Why humans might have traded this approach [hunting-gathering] for the complexities of agriculture is an interesting and long-debated question, especially because the skeletal evidence clearly indicates that early farmers were more poorly nourished, more disease-ridden, and deformed, than their hunter-gatherer contemporaries.*[6]

The original hunter-gatherers ate everything in their ecosystems that was digestible, from raw soil laden with organic material and microorganisms (South American indigenous peoples) to the stomach contents of freshly slain bison (Native Americans of the Plains states). The Inuits of Alaska consumed a huge proportion of protein and fat from fish and seal blubber, and a smaller amount of complex plant carbohydrates. Pacific Island hunter-gatherers ate predominantly the protein and fats of fish, and a greater proportion of complex carbohydrates from plants—coconut, taro root, some fruits, nuts, and seeds. In Papua New Guinea, diets centered on animal protein, fats, and plant products, but fats were again prized. African forest Aka Pygmies relied on plant products for only one-third of their diet, and meat and fat for the remainder. The geographically nearby G/wi and G//ana of Botswana consumed complex carbohydrates for 80 percent of the diet, including tubers, melons, truffles, nuts, and lilies, while scarcer meat made up only 20 percent of the diet.

Three important lessons emerge already from this brief survey of hunter-gatherer diets, and help us reconstruct a modern integrated diet (figure 10.1). First, our distant ancestors weren't fussy about what they ate. Food was precious and scarce biological fuel, and they used every edible portion of every plant and animal they could find in their ecosystem. A possible lesson: Avoid seduction by the taste or flavor of food, which may not be the best indicator of whether it is useful as a valuable source of biological energy.

A second possible lesson from hunter-gatherer diets is that food variety across and between groups was enormous. There were as many diets as there were hunter-gatherer peoples, and our genes are therefore unprepared for a one-size-fits-all diet. The third possible lesson is historic reliance on local and seasonal availability. Hunter-gatherers ate whatever they could find in their bioregion, and natural selection fine-tuned the local gene pool accordingly.

FIGURE 10.1
THE INTEGRATED DIET

Hunter-gatherer diets show what nature prepared us to eat today. On that basis, we can identify a dozen principles of the integrated diet:

1. **Food is biological fuel.** Design your diet accordingly.

2. **Eat a varied diet.** That is how you get all the diverse fuel you need.

3. **There is no single ideal diet.** Find yours by self-experimentation, with body consciousness as your tool.

4. **Emphasize bioregional and seasonal foods.** Many modern people retain ties to ancestral ecosystems in which their genes evolved, and consuming bioregional foods conserves resources.

5. **Fat is essential.** Make fats 35 percent of your diet (40 percent for kids), and eat mostly unsaturated fats (such as olive oil) and uncontaminated fish fats, but with regular exercise.

6. **Complex carbohydrates are essential.** Make them up to 65 percent of your diet, and get them mainly from vegetables and whole grains.

7. **Protein is essential.** It need make up no more than 25 percent of your diet, however, and can come safely from plant sources if you choose.

8. **Exclude refined sugar.** It contributes to many of the modern illnesses, including obesity, metabolic syndrome, and diabetes.

9. **Limit simple carbohydrates.** Your body doesn't need them as fuel, and is not prepared for them genetically.

10. **Avoid processed, refined, and preserved foods.** Read labels and avoid preservatives. Daily ingestion of poison is unhealthy.

11. **Eat organic food whenever possible.** Evolution didn't prepare us to eat poisonous pesticides and herbicides, and they damage the earth.

12. **Eat lightly and well.** You will live a longer, healthier, happier life!

Throughout most of human history, physical barriers such as mountains and oceans, combined with the difficulty of traveling long distances, confined most people to the ecosystem where they were born. The thousands of tribes of Papua New Guinea, for example, were so isolated from one another that they developed thousands of distinct languages, of which 4,000—one-third of the world's total—still exist. A few years ago, scientists used DNA fingerprinting to identify a man living in a small English village who was a direct genetic descendant of a fossilized Stone Age hunter found nearby from 8,000 years earlier. Nature had plenty of time to emblazon local diets into human genetics, and science is just starting to identify the genetic mutations that optimized survival in unique or extreme ecosystems.

Metabolic Typing

Although our genes originally contained the indelible dietary stamp of a specific ecosystem, modern transportation permits many of us to live far from our original ecosystem. Modern transportation also makes foods from different ecosystems available to many, and enables mixing genes with those of people from entirely different genetic backgrounds. Some people with genotypes close to the original, such as Native Americans and other indigenous peoples, may still find reliable dietary guidance from ancestral diets. The rest of us, however, must experiment to find out our most advantageous diet, using trial and error based on informed choice, dietary preference, and physiological response.

This is not a new idea. William Wolcott, author of *The Metabolic Typing Diet*, noted that our ancestors developed a genetic predisposition to thrive on certain food types. The secret to the right diet for each person lies encrypted in our own genes, and all we have to do is decode it. You can find your optimum integrated diet by observing your weight and body composition, your allergic reactions (if any), your emotions, and your physical sensations. Pay close attention to the seasons, as hunter-gatherers did—for what works in winter may not work in summer. The same body consciousness you use for your IBC workout is your primary tool in the quest for your optimum integrated diet.

Fats Are Essential

One of the most remarkable features of the hunter-gatherers' diets was how much fat they contained. In many hunter-gatherer societies, complex plant carbohydrates were a supplemental food source. The main food was protein and fat. Blackfoot Indians of the American Plains rendered bison carcasses for pure fat, which they stored as pemmican. A high-fat diet did not harm the health of hunter-gatherers—they did not suffer from high cholesterol, coronary disease, or diabetes, which are all modern diseases. Contrary to conventional wisdom, the hunter-gatherers' diet and lifestyle kept them alive for at least as long as us. Average life expectancy is higher now, but that's because child mortality has decreased, extending the *average* length of a human life. The eldest hunter-gatherers were little different in age from the eldest moderns.

The hunter-gatherer's diet raises two dietary paradoxes, one medical and one biological. The medical paradox is that hunter-gatherers evidently lived to a ripe old age on a high-fat diet, yet modern medical authorities advise us to limit fat intake. Diets high in saturated fats do increase coronary risk in modern people. The biological paradox is that fat, in the form of phospholipids, is the building material for the membranous skeleton and skin of every cell in our body. If so much of our body is made of fat, and if that fat is available only from our diet, why is a high-fat diet apparently harmful to modern people?

Both the medical and the biological paradox could have the same solution: integrated exercise. As we saw earlier (chapter 2), hunter-gatherer people worked hard physically just to survive. Modern people, as we know, don't get enough exercise of any kind. The problem may not be eating too much fat, but getting too little exercise. Medical research is starting to confirm this view. A recent study divided 127 Finnish men into four groups, and examined the relation between dietary fat intake, physical fitness, and blood concentrations of harmful fat products. Dietary intake of fats was the same in all groups, but the researchers discovered that the blood levels of unhealthy saturated fatty acids were lower, and healthy polyunsaturated fats higher, in the most physically fit group. Saturated fat intake in the diet was associated with high blood levels of saturated fats only in the least fit group.

Apparently, people who exercise are less vulnerable to harmful effects of dietary fat. This conclusion receives support from studies showing that a single bout of exercise increases the body's use of dietary fat from a recent meal. These and other findings suggest that the key to health and weight control is not in avoiding fat, but rather in exercising. As long as you get plenty of exercise—as hunter-gatherers did—you can apparently consume some fats with some abandon, because the liver and muscles use them rapidly for energy and cellular construction.

There is, however, a qualification to the suggestion that we can consume fats with abandon. Many toxins found in the modern environment are lipophilic—they dissolve in fat and are stored there for constant release into our blood. When we consume fat from nonorganic sources, such as commercially available beef and pork, we also ingest whatever toxins their feed contained. That is enough reason to eat organic food, including meat. A happier, disease-free life and lower medical bills more than compensate the extra cost. Fish and fish fat are among the healthiest foods you can eat. Most fish, and particularly fish fat, however, is now contaminated with mercury and PCBs, to the level that even the U.S. government issues regular warnings to limit consumption. Fortunately, you can still get clean, organic fish, and fish oil, from Dr. Mercola through his website (www.mercola. com). The National Academy of Sciences (NAS) 2002 Dietary Reference Standard does not establish a daily intake level of saturated fats, which are solid at room temperature, because they have no known benefits in preventing chronic disease. It does suggest using unsaturated fats, which are liquid at room temperature, as much as possible to lower blood cholesterol and heart disease.

Carbohydrates and the Low-Carb Craze

How should we moderns balance protein/fat and carbohydrates in our diets? The late Dr. Robert Atkins believed that we eat far too many carbohydrates, and far more than nature intended, making it hard to lose weight. It is a good point, and utilizes the same logic invoked to support IBC. The Atkins diet runs aground, however, on some well-established dietary science (see the sidebar on page 222).

Our primary source of muscle energy, glycogen, is a complex carbohydrate synthesized from carbohydrates in our diet. If we do not eat enough carbohydrates, the body obtains energy by breaking down muscle tissue. That's a great adaptation for survival in hard times, but no way to build muscle. In extreme cases, a low-carbohydrate diet can reduce lean tissue mass and overwork the kidneys by flooding them with urea and other products of protein metabolism.

Moreover, the metabolic products of carbohydrate breakdown are themselves essential priming agents for burning fat. Contrary to the most basic premise of the Atkins diet, carbohydrates contribute to weight loss. Eliminate carbohydrates from your diet and you deprive yourself of one of the most important metabolic tools available to shed fat while preserving muscle. As exercise professionals put it, if you want to lose weight, "burn fat in a carbohydrate flame."

Why do so many people swear by the Atkins diet, and actually lose weight when they follow it? The answer comes in two parts, one obvious and one less so. The obvious answer is that carbohydrates compose about half the total calories in the typical American diet, and half of all carbohydrate intake is simple sugars—refined sugar, sucrose, and high-fructose corn or rice syrup. That translates to a yearly intake of 60 pounds of table sugar and 46 pounds of syrup; in contrast, our grandparents ingested only 4 pounds of sugar per year, and they did not suffer from obesity and the related metabolic diseases nearly to the same extent. People lose weight on the Atkins diet

because they cannot indulge in 400-calorie bagels, 600-calorie muffins, Krispy Kreme doughnuts, Häagen-Dazs ice cream, pies, cakes, cookies or even rice, pasta, bread or potatoes. Nor can they grab a candy bar or down a sugary soda when the snack bug bites.[7]

A calorie is a calorie no matter where it comes from, and 3,500 extra calories make a pound of fat.

The less obvious reason that people on a low-carbohydrate diet shed weight initially has to do with how the body stores biological energy. Carbohydrates are the main source of internal glycogen, which is the primary—and fastest—source of energy for both muscle and brain. Each pound of glycogen that your body holds is bound up with 2.7 pounds of water. Eliminate carbohydrates from your diet, and you reduce glycogen; reduce glycogen, and you shed more than twice the poundage in the form of water. In other words, the initial weight loss from a low-carbohydrate diet is not fat, but water.

The Atkins and South Beach low-carbohydrate diets do shed pounds, but not for the reasons most people think. From a biological perspective, eliminating carbohydrates from your diet is a mistake because carbohydrates:

- Are the best source of biological energy even if you are trying to lose weight.
- Protect muscle tissue from being destroyed for energy.
- Prime your metabolism for fat loss, because their metabolites light the fires that burn fat.
- Provide the best metabolic support for high-intensity exercise because they produce glycogen, which supplies power more directly and twice as fast as energy from fat or protein.
- Feed your brain best with their ultimate breakdown product, glucose, the main fuel for the brain.

These carbohydrate facts may explain the result of a study published in the January 2004 edition of the *Annals of Internal Medicine* in which people on a high-carbohydrate diet readily lost weight. Weight loss occurs whenever you burn more calories than you eat, regardless of whether your diet is rich or sparse in carbohydrates. The best way to lose weight is not to eliminate carbohydrates, but instead to exercise more to ignite your metabolism through exercise, consume no more calories than you burn, and make sure your diet is integrated (figure 10.1).

Good and Bad Carbohydrates

Not all carbohydrates, however, are beneficial. To identify the good ones—those that evolution prepared us to utilize best—we need look no further than the "gatherer" part of the hunter-gatherer's diet. Our ancestors collected and consumed

Myth Buster 10: The Low-Carb Craze

THE MYTH: Low-carb diets can help me lose fat and stay healthy.

Diets that restrict carbohydrates have changed the landscape of the modern dinner table, spawning a whole new product line of low-carb foods, beer, and even vitamin supplements for the low-carb diet. Atkins Inc. is a $100 million business, and *The South Beach Diet* has sold millions of copies. Numerous Americans have voted with their pocketbooks and now pursue low-carb diets in a misguided search for weight loss and health. And many lose weight, at least initially, reinforcing the illusion that they are on the right track.

Carbohydrate is the main source of energy that fuels muscle contraction, glycogen. Every gram of glycogen in the body binds to 2.7 grams of water. When you reduce your carbohydrate intake, you also reduce internal stores of glycogen, which releases the water. That initial weight loss is nothing more than a rapid loss of the water that is normally bound to glycogen. And that, unfortunately, is just the beginning of the problems with a low-carb diet.

You actually need carbs to lose fat! The metabolic burning of fatty acids depends on a continual background level of metabolites from carbohydrate breakdown, particularly one called oxaloacetate. That's why exercise professionals say if you want to lose weight without losing muscle, "burn fat in a carbo flame." Take away the carbs, and you deprive yourself of a powerful tool for true fat loss, as opposed to dehydration masquerading as fat loss.

Carbs spare muscle by reducing protein catabolism. Carbohydrate is also your main energy source during high-intensity exercise. Limit your carb intake and try to exercise vigorously, and you'll feel the fatigue. Fat takes up some slack, but muscles burn fat at only half the rate of carbs, so your power is limited. Carbs are also your main source of glucose, which is the main fuel used by the brain. Cut carbs, and your brain has no choice but to turn to fats, which causes brain fatigue. In other words, a low-carb diet dramatically reduces your physical and mental power. And if you are on a low-carb diet and don't notice the fatigue, that's a sign you are operating at too low a capacity to challenge your system.

THE REALITY: Low-carb diets inhibit fat loss and restrict physical and mental capacity.

The IBC Myth Buster

MYTH: Low-carb diets help lose weight and are healthy.

FACT: At least half of a healthy diet should come from complex carbohydrates.

mainly complex carbohydrates—roots and tubers, seeds and nuts, fungi, acorns, and berries. Since we still have their genes, complex carbohydrates are the most beneficial to us, too. Because these carbohydrates are complex, our metabolism takes time to break them down, so they supply slow, steady energy to replenish glycogen stores. That in turn moderates and spares our insulin reactions, protecting from metabolic diseases such as diabetes.

Consumption of such good carbohydrates has the additional advantage of providing all the fiber and most of the vitamins required for the integrated diet. Fiber is the nonstarch structural element of plants that is largely lost through refining and processing foods. High fiber intake confers lower incidence of heart disease, obesity, and high blood pressure, among other benefits. Sources include whole oats, bran, peas and beans, apples, potatoes, and broccoli—all complex carbohydrates. The National Academy of Sciences Dietary Reference Standard recommends different amounts of fiber for different age groups, ranging from 21 grams (about 0.75 ounce) for women over 50, to 38 grams (a little over an ounce) for younger men. The regular consumption of unprocessed complex carbohydrates easily provides these recommended daily amounts.

The hunter-gatherer diet is illuminating, however, not only for what it contained, but also for what it lacked. No hunter-gatherer people anywhere on earth evolved eating refined sugar—a simple carbohydrate that may be the single most destructive component of the modern diet. When modern civilization introduces sugar to the diet of hunter-gatherers, the results are disastrous. In the tiny Pacific island nation of Nauru, for example, canned foods, soft drinks, and alcohol have displaced the traditional diet of fish, coconut, and taro root. Almost all adults are overweight or obese; two-thirds are diabetic, and the average life span is less than 50 years and declining. The people of Nauru may provide a brief history of our own future: The U.S. Centers for Disease Control in Atlanta warns us that one of three children born in the year 2000 in the United States will become diabetic unless there is a radical evolution of dietary consciousness and an increase in exercise. The lesson is clear: Eliminate refined sugar from your diet.

Simple carbohydrates such as sugars are clearly harmful, but there are also two forms of complex carbohydrates that can be problematic—alcohol and grains. Small amounts of alcohol can be beneficial. The risk of coronary heart disease drops by nearly half with a couple of glasses of red wine per day, though it increases again with more drinks. Red wine contains a chemical—resveratrol—known from animal studies to prolong life (see below). Alcohol contains 7 calories per gram, however, and is therefore nearly as fattening as fat (9 calories per gram). A single ounce of pure alcohol contains around 250 calories, and those two drinks that furnish heart protection therefore contain more than 10 percent of a typical recommended daily caloric intake. Alcohol can be a diet buster. Moreover, as we will see below, the heart-protective effects of resveratrol may be obtainable in a much easier, diet-friendly, and alcohol-free way—by eating less.

The second complex carbohydrate that may be problematic for modern people is grain. Our hunter-gatherer ancestors did not get many carbohydrates from grains because the biomass of grain foods available in nature was small in relation to other complex plant carbohydrates such as roots and tubers. The typical hunter-gatherer diet probably contained less than 10 percent grains—largely wild wheat, rice, and later cultivated maize (corn)—which found use primarily as a carbohydrate supplement. In contrast, today only two cultivated grains—wheat and rice—supply an estimated 60 percent of all "direct" human calories.

The massive influx of grains into the human diet provides a challenge to the human genotype, which is unprepared for so radical a change in such short evolutionary time. Dr. Joseph Mercola suggests that overconsumption of grains contributes to many modern nutritional and dietary allergies and diseases, including diabetes and obesity. The Mercola No-Grain diet does not propose the elimination of grains, however. Instead, it incorporates individual variation in diet response and proposes a calibration of your response to dietary grain employing a form of body consciousness.

How much carbohydrate do we need every day to maintain health? The National Academy of Sciences Dietary Reference Standard of 2002 recommends 130 grams of carbohydrates a day for children and adults for adequate brain function. That's about 520 calories a day, or around 30 percent of the calories required for an average person. Physically active people and athletes, however, need up to twice that proportion—60 percent or more of the total diet in the form of carbohydrates—to support their healthy habits.

Protein: Enough Is Enough

The Atkins and South Beach diets suggest that proteins and fats together should make up the bulk of our diet. Our survey of the hunter-gatherer diet, however, suggests that our genes are prepared for a diet consisting of no more than half fats and proteins. Your body requires less protein than you might think, even if you are an elite athlete. Too much protein can put a strain on your system, because the breakdown products, including urea and other metabolites, are hard on the liver and kidneys. Too much protein can therefore impose a physiological cost without a corresponding benefit.

According to the U.S. National Academy of Sciences, the recommended level of protein intake of a physically active nonathlete adult is 0.8 gram per kilogram of body weight, or about a hundredth of an ounce per pound of body weight. A 200-pound man therefore needs only 75 grams of protein a day, around 3 ounces, to meet normal metabolic requirements. In terms of calories, that is about 15 percent of total dietary intake. If 30 percent of our dietary intake is fats, and at least 50 percent is carbohydrates, that leaves only 20 percent for proteins anyway—plenty for the "average" diet, although you can adjust that to your individual circumstances.

Only pregnant women and athletes in extremely heavy training—two to six hours per day of vigorous resistance exercise, like Olympic athletes—need consider increasing their protein intake. The NAS Dietary Reference Standard suggests that pregnant women consume 25 grams—a little less than an ounce—a day above their nonpregnant intake level. Standards for athletes in heavy training have not been determined. Pending the necessary research, exercise professionals recommend consumption of 1.2–1.8 grams of protein per kilogram of body mass daily. The high end of this recommended range corresponds to an extra 2 ounces a day for a 200-pound athlete, for a total daily intake of around 4 ounces per day of protein—equivalent to a quarter pound of lean meat or a few eggs.

Dietary Risks and How to Avoid Them

Refined sugar is not the only component of the modern diet that was absent from the diet of hunter-gatherers. Hunter-gatherers ate no highly processed foods, and no preservatives, which are in reality metabolic poisons added mainly to extend shelf life. Hunter-gatherers ate no white bread stripped of nutrition and bleached with chlorine for appearance, very little grain, no highly glycemic foods such as certain modern fruits, no pesticides, no herbicides, and no genetically modified foods. Our genes are unprepared for every one of these increasingly widespread components of the modern human diet.

The simplest and healthiest way to avoid these harmful dietary components is to eat whole organic foods. Dr. Dean Edell cites five studies on the nutritional profile of organic foods, four of which allegedly showed no difference and one of which showed a superior nutritional profile for organic foods. Our hunter-gatherer ancestors certainly ate organic, leaving our genes unprepared for synthetic pesticides. Even if pesticides posed no more than a minor risk to human health from ingestion, their use concentrates them in ecosystems to pose a threat to many forms of animal life. DDT came close to exterminating the bald eagle and the brown pelican, and related toxins continue to wreak the damage that Rachel Carson prophesied decades ago.

An integrated perspective, one that incorporates interconnectedness, invites equal concern for our own bodies and the earth that sustains us. If we're in fact part of the same system, then anything that hurts one endangers the other. Even if the jury is still out on nutritional advantages of organic food, choose them whenever possible to protect your own health and the health of the planet.

Hunter-gatherers offer yet another dietary lesson. Food was so hard to find, prepare, and store that they ate very little and burned every calorie they consumed. Consequently, they were almost never overweight or obese. Research conducted by the late Dr. Roy Walford and his colleagues at UCLA showed that mice fed a 50 percent calorie-restricted diet live twice as long. Research on geese, dogs, and monkeys has yielded similar findings.

What is the cause of the apparent benefit of eating lightly? Calorie-restricted diets produce in the bodies of these animals resveratrol—that same "fountain of youth" chemical (technically a polyphenolic bioflavonoid) found in red wine. Researchers at Harvard Medical School showed recently that the same chemical extends the life span of yeast and fruit flies. No one has yet done the research to establish that this works in people, although the U.S. government is reportedly investing millions of dollars in research funds for that purpose. In the meantime, the President's Council on Bioethics cautions that

> the pursuit of an ageless body [through calorie-restriction diets] may prove finally to be a distraction and a deformation.[8]

Hunter-gatherers' diets may contain a final lesson, this one about vitamins. There is a multibillion-dollar industry based on the idea that we don't get everything we need from our normal diet and therefore should take vitamins and minerals, and even amino acids, among other things. There are an estimated 500,000 supplement products on the market, created by 2,500 manufacturers, with an annual gross of $1.9 billion. Pick up any fitness magazine, and you will find that the majority of advertisements are for supplements. Do they work, are they necessary, and are they worth the substantial cost?

Hunter-gatherers did not use supplements; they got everything they needed from their diet. From an evolutionary and genetic viewpoint, therefore, supplements are suspect. They are also suspect from a scientific viewpoint—the vast majority of supplements lack scientific support, and the companies themselves generally produce the limited science that is available. Supplements are also suspect from the perspective of the drug industry culture. The U.S. Food and Drug Administration (FDA) regulates pharmaceuticals, but supplements escape the same regulation, owing to the 1994 Dietary Supplement Health and Education Act. This federal legislation gave consumers access to alternative health and medical remedies, but, like many government policies, it also had a very different and unforeseen effect. Following the adoption of this legislation at the national level, there was a virtual explosion of athletic supplement products. Legislation intended to increase consumer choice thus ended up fueling an explosion in unproven dietary supplements.

Vitamins are the best-known and bestselling supplements. Most nutritional experts, however, are convinced they're unnecessary if you are eating a varied and healthy diet. Vitamin E supplementation does reduce the concentration of free radicals (oxidants) in the body, but vitamin E is also one of the fat-soluble vitamins (including A, D, and K) that can be harmful or toxic in excess. Some clinical evidence suggests that folic acid counters aspects of cardiovascular disease. In addition, iron may be advisable, under some circumstances, for menstruating women, but excess iron is also toxic. All of these vitamins and minerals, however, come in a healthy, varied, and balanced diet. Nutrition author and professor Shawn Talbott of the University of Utah described the diet supplement industry as "pretty much the Wild West."[9]

Even if we don't need vitamins, can they enhance performance? More than 50 percent of athletes surveyed in one study said they took vitamin supplements, and research shows that vitamin supplementation by elite athletes exceeds that of college athletes, which exceeds that of high school athletes. The research also suggests, however, that there is no performance advantage. The Australia Institute of Sport recently evaluated 82 elite athletes in four sports: swimming, rowing, gymnastics, and basketball. The athletes who took vitamins showed no measurable improvement in any sport. Indeed, the only measurable effect was increased blood and urine levels of the ingested vitamins. A recent review on the topic of vitamin supplementation concluded that

> the number of studies with rigorous methods standards from which firm conclusions may be drawn is few, while the intensity of the marketing and promotion of most nutritional supplements is intense and far exceeds the data supporting their use.[10]

An exercise physiology text sums it up this way.

> Over 40 years of research does not support using vitamin supplements to improve exercise performance or ability to train arduously in nutritionally adequate healthy people. . . . The sale of vitamins is probably the biggest rip-off in our society today. Their only effect would appear to be a highly enriched sewage around athletic training or competition sites.[11]

How about those popular protein powders that are offered as muscle builders? You get all the protein your body can use from a few ounces of meat each day and/or a few eggs, even if you are an athlete in heavy training or a menstruating woman. Moreover, many protein supplements are harmful because they have high concentrations of simple amino acids that the intestinal wall cannot absorb well and that can cause dehydration.

> *The common practice among weight lifters, body builders, and other power athletes of consuming liquids, powders, or pills of predigested protein represents a waste of money and may actually be counterproductive for producing the desired outcome."*[12]

Do you need "electrolyte-replacing" drinks or "health bars" to replenish energy? Unless you run daily marathons, or exercise for long periods in high heat and humidity, you easily replace all your electrolytes with a sound diet. "Health bars" are not nearly as healthy as the industry would like us to believe. They typically contain high-fructose corn syrup, or concentrated fruit juices high in fructose, as their "natural" sweetener. Research shows that fructose is worse for test animals than refined sugar. In addition, the protein contained in "health bars" is often derived from soybeans. Soy protein is coming under scrutiny by researchers, who point out that soy contains phytoestrogens that mimic the effects of the normal female hormone estrogen. Two glasses of soy milk a day can alter a woman's menstrual cycle, and infants fed on soy formula receive the equivalent of five birth control pills' worth of estrogen every day.

A small carbohydrate supplement every two or three hours can be helpful during long bouts of intensive training (more than two hours), restoring and sustaining blood glucose. "Health bars," however, are not the healthiest choice. Following your workout, replenish your fuel source as soon as practicable by consuming carbohydrate-rich foods. Even under ideal circumstances, however, your body can regenerate only about 5 percent of your glycogen fuel supply per hour, so you may not fully recover, energetically, for up to 20 hours after a heavy workout.

Drugs

Many supplements bill themselves as "performance enhancers." In some cases, such as that of anabolic steroids, they can cause biological and psychological harm that outweighs any potential health or short-term performance benefit. Decades ago, scientists discovered that steroids increase muscle mass and strength, and some trainers and some sports doctors prescribed them for athletes. The effects of steroids are nonspecific, however. The "side effects" range from cardiovascular and liver damage, brain malfunction, mood and personality disorders, to shorter lives—just the opposite from the health and wellness goals that exercise should achieve.

The latest drug craze for building muscle is creatine. According to theory, it could shore up your short-term phosphorus energy system and give your muscles a more explosive and enduring "first gear," thus amplifying the training effects of exercise—and there is ample scientific evidence that creatine increases muscle mass and strength. Knowing that the body is an interacting system, however, cautions that creatine affects not just muscle, but also brain and liver, gonad and gut. The "side effects" on other tissues and organs, and for that matter on muscle, are still a mystery, just as the "side effects" of steroids were unknown in the 1950s. Creatine supplementation could also undermine the natural response to exercise by depriving muscles of the opportunity to accelerate their own energy replenishment systems naturally through training.

Drug scandals abound in athletics. The latest involves the San Francisco Bay Area Laboratory Co-Operative, which allegedly supplied a number of high-profile trainers and athletes with the new "designer steroid" tetrahydrogestrinone. The scandal has touched professional baseball and football, and reached clear to the 2004 Summer Olympics, illustrating how widespread the drug epidemic is among elite athletes. It's a hard game to beat—as soon as scientists find a way to detect a particular drug, enterprising drug dealers find a way to disguise it so it can't be detected with conventional or easy biochemical techniques. Children get the message and turn increasingly to whatever "performance-enhancing substances" they can find. And they are not hard to find. A California survey released in March 2004 by the office of the governor indicated that half of high school boys, and a third of high school girls, knew someone who took anabolic steroids—mainly to "look good."

The corruption by drugs of such a noble endeavor as human athletics understandably saddens and outrages many people. Unfortunately, the reliance on drugs is in part a reflection of the general acceptance of drugs in Western culture and medicine. Watch the evening news, and count the number of advertisements for drugs designed and marketed to improve human performance by dealing with issues from illness and allergies to heartburn and impotence. The Western medical approach often de-emphasizes the cause and instead seeks a chemical fix to ameliorate the effect. Western medicine and the American medical community are key players in this drug culture, and we, the consumers, are participants.

Economics untempered by ethics drives this behavior, in sports and in our culture at large. All athletes are at risk because the slightest performance boost can translate into tens of thousands of dollars in salary and bonuses, fame, and status. When athletes and kids turn to drugs for "performance enhancement" or a muscled look, however, they reflect our culture back to us. The ethical issues surrounding drugs in exercise therefore go deeper than sports—we need to reevaluate our cultural and medical attitudes to drugs in general. As Charles Yesalis and Michael Bahrke have observed,

> *It is our society that emphasizes and rewards speed, strength, size, aggressiveness and, above all, winning. Thus, the behavior of athletes and sports officials in the matter of doping is congruent with their customers' desires.*[13]

When society rejects the use of performance-enhancing drugs across the board, athletes will be more likely to follow suit. Pending such a change in cultural paradigm, education, rigorous drug testing, and severe penalties for violations appear to be the main options.

Sleep Well

Sleep is at least as important as diet in any exercise regimen for most people. We're getting less of it, however, in comparison with our recent ancestors. Americans sleep an average of seven hours a night, compared with eight hours for our parents' generation, and ten hours for our great-grandparents. The lack of sleep is one of the many reasons for rising stress in modern society.

Lack of sleep may impact strongly on exercise. Both of my bonks in the last two years (chapter 6) occurred after insufficient sleep, and at least two athletes I have trained showed elevated heart rates—up to 25 percent above normal—following travel-related sleep deprivation. These limited observations don't constitute a scientific study, and I'm not aware of any research on the topic. There is, however, strong scientific reason for believing that sleep might disrupt the normal exercise response, related to the biological clock.

The human brain contains a biological clock that ticks away on a near-24-hour rhythm and entrains every cell in our body with its signal—the circadian rhythm. The master clock is a small knot of neurons immediately above the hypothalamus, called the suprachiasmatic nucleus. This biological clock regulates every facet of our metabolism, including energy conversion and heart rate. The clock can be disrupted easily—phase shifted, in scientific parlance—by a single night of disrupted or insufficient sleep, or by switching rapidly to a different time zone (jet lag). Disrupting our biological clock changes the metabolism of our muscles, including our heart, which could affect the response to exercise. Disrupted or insufficient sleep is also a well-established cause of depression and can even trigger bipolar disorders such as manic-depressive behavior and other psychological problems.

That same biological clock gets confused if you retire and awaken at different times each day. Imagine what would happen to your body's band if the rhythm, string, and brass sections all played at different tempos. Now imagine that happening throughout your whole body. Interrupt your circadian rhythm, even for a day, and you can become physiologically dis-integrated until your clock gets reset—and that can be disastrous for exercise performance. The advice we all got from Mom or Dad still works: Keep a regular bedtime and get enough sleep—eight hours every night for most people. If for any reason you cannot get enough sleep, or are jet lagged, skip your workout or step down its intensity until your biorhythms get resynchronized.

A Miracle Workout World

Systems theory implies that our physical condition depends in part on our culture. Obesity is not just a matter of exercising too little or eating too much—it is also a matter of frenetic, unbalanced, fragmented, sedentary, and stressful lives. Errant public policies don't help—refined sugar and genetically modified foods have been subsidized for years by the U.S. government, and schools routinely install vending machines to distribute these products to our children. Corporate policies haven't helped—soft drink companies spend $500 million every year to advertise their sugary sodas. In contrast, the advertising budgets for fruits and vegetables are closer to a million a year. The companies are in the business of producing whatever we will buy, however, so ultimately it is up to us, the consumers, to make informed choices and teach our children to do the same.

The increasing severity of the obesity epidemic and related illnesses, combined with the escalating cost of health care and the fact that 45 million Americans lack health insurance, has intensified the debate, which some call "the great American food fight."[14] Should exercise and diet be a personal concern and responsibility, or a social agenda, or both? One side argues that government can and should use its legislative power to help educate and slim down the American population. Obesity, like smoking, is a social problem with social and economic costs that you and I pay with hard-earned tax dollars. The other side argues that the government should not legislate eating or exercise behaviors, which are matters of personal choice and responsibility.

Both views have merit, but perhaps the question itself is wrong, in that it sets up a false dichotomy. Exercising and eating well *are* a personal choice, in that they affect individual lives. They are equally a social issue, however, because they have such a powerful impact on the well-being of society. Perhaps the solution could come at both levels. IBC can serve as a solution at the personal level, and if it were supported at the social level, it could make for a happier, more productive, more self-efficacious population and workforce. Finland has pioneered public policies and programs encouraging healthy food and exercise habits among its people, and it's working. The question is not who should properly address this massive and growing individual and social problem in America, nor whether or even when. The real question is *how*.

Consider American elementary schools, where the relentless emphasis on academic achievement combined with the budget crunch has deprioritized physical education. Exercise conditions both the body and the brain, however; as we have seen, people are better at mental tasks when the physical body is healthy and well conditioned. If higher test scores and scholastic achievement represent the desired end, then the means must surely include healthful food and exercise at school, as well as education in both. It would be easy to build integrated exercise into an elementary school routine—just provide enough organized and supervised playtime and play space each day, and the kids will take care of the rest.

By the time children reach high school, many have attained a measure of maturity that could support more systematic, integrated exercise programs. For an outdoor IBC workout, run them up the stairs of the football bleachers for cardio conditioning and cardio-acceleration. Then, while their heart rates are elevated, turn them loose for sets of ROM and multijoint barbell and dumbbell resistance exercises, or simply push-ups and curl-ups. On rainy days, set up the high school gym with inexpensive jump ropes, step-up boxes, or Bosu Balls for cardio-acceleration, with the weights on nearby mats. Combine these activities with education about diet, exercise, and health, and put it into action by getting rid of vending machines that ply students with candy, chips, and soft drinks. Sound and practical high school education in diet and integrated exercise could help put children on a path to health and wellness that would last a lifetime, and help relieve enormous looming personal and social strain on the larger society.

Graduation to college is another of those vulnerable passages (chapter 8) that can alter the course of life. I have taught a Discovery Seminar in exercise physiology at the University of California that integrates students into our research program on IBC, and students say it made all the difference in their college experience and their attitude toward exercise. Exercise also makes all the difference in the university's bottom line—retention is up to 25 percent higher for students who participate in athletic programs. Every college or university could benefit by building exercise and diet programs to help its incoming students get on the right track. It's not only fun, but is also in the best interests of the whole university community.

Can regular exercise work in the workplace? Just ask the pharmaceutical company Hoffmann–La Roche, the appliance maker Whirlpool, the health care giant Johnson & Johnson, Parker Hannifin Corporation, or Sprint, among others. These are some of the corporate leaders that have initiated exercise programs at work, not just to make happier workers (which is working), but also to help them become more productive and save enormously on health and medical costs—and therefore contribute to the corporate bottom line. According to a recent study in *Health Affairs,* the cost of obesity alone to U.S. business could top $30 billion a year, and it's growing. When we add the costs to the 45 million uninsured Americans, the added strains on the creaking U.S. health care system, and the increasing stresses on Social Security, Medicare, and related health care programs, and when we consider the aging U.S. population—the total cost could eventually eclipse the national budget deficit!

The question is not whether it is the government's job to make Americans exercise and slim down. The question is, in view of what we can plainly see happening, what are we waiting for? There are socially acceptable and cost-effective ways to educate and encourage Americans, and indeed people all over the world, to eat right and exercise. Health and wellness are the sine qua non of civilization and the fountainhead of human potential. Integrated diets and exercise are in the interests of all, from the individual to society to the whole of modern civilization. Unless we start immediately, it is not clear that our health and welfare system can absorb the additional weight without cracking.

It's not yet too late. All it takes is integrated thinking, an integrated lifestyle, and integrated exercise, at every level, for all. What have we got to lose but a few pounds and a bushel of misery? What we may have to gain is the fuller realization of human potential in our time.

Chapter 1: The Integrated Exercise Revolution

1. William D. McArdle, Frank I. Katch, and Victor L. Katch. *Essentials of Exercise Physiology,* second edition (Philadelphia: Lippincott Williams & Wilkins, 2000), p. 593.

Chapter 2: The Art of the Miracle Workout

1. www.mercola.com/2003/aug/23/alzheimers.htm.
2. Gina Kolata. *Ultimate Fitness: The Quest for Truth About Exercise and Health* (New York: Farrar, Straus and Giroux, 2003), p. 183.
3. Ibid., p. 180.
4. Ibid., p. 148.
5. Ibid., p. 184.
6. R. G. Holly and J. D. Shaffrath. "Cardiorespiratory Endurance." In American College of Sports Medicine. *ACSM's Resource Manual for Guidelines for Exercise Testing and Prescription,* fourth edition (Philadelphia: Lippincott Williams & Wilkins, 2001), p. 458.

Chapter 3: The Science of the Miracle Workout

1. Arnold Schwarzenegger. "Clue in to Cardio." *Muscle Fitness* (June 2003), p. 192.
2. Aida Leisenring. "Is Cardio Dead?" *Elle* (2003), p. 34.

Chapter 6: Your Advanced Miracle Workout

1. Jane E. Brody. "A Pregame Ritual: Doctors Averting Disasters." *The New York Times* (October 14, 2003), p. D7.
2. A. Verghese. "Pain Gains." *The New York Times Magazine* (July 27, 2003), p. 10.

Chapter 7: Do What You Love

1. J. Larry Durstine, J. L. Davis, and Paul G. Davis. "Specificity of Exercise Training and Testing." In American College of Sports Medicine. *ACSM's Resource Manual for Guidelines for Exercise Testing and Prescription,* fourth edition (Philadelphia: Lippincott Williams & Wilkins, 2001), chapter 56, p. 489.

2. L. Ruzic, S. Heimer, M. Misigoj-Durakovic, and B. R. Matkovic. "Increased Occupational Physical Activity Does Not Improve Physical Fitness." *Occup Environ Med* 60 (2003), pp. 983–985.

Chapter 8: Stay in the Game

1. Franz Kafka. *The Collected Aphorisms* (New York: Penguin, 1994), translated by M. Pasley.
2. National Academy of Sciences, Food and Nutrition Board, Institute of Medicine. *Dietary Reference Intakes for Energy, Carbohydrate, Fiber, Fat, Fatty Acids, Cholesterol, Protein and Amino Acids (Macronutrients)* (Washington, D.C.: National Academy of Sciences Press, 2002), p. 12–1. Available free online at www.nap.edu.
3. Ibid.

Chapter 9: Special Populations and Conditions

1. Team Physician Consensus Statement. "Female Athlete Issues for the Team Physician: A Consensus Statement." Special Communications, *Med Sci Sports Exer* (2003), pp. 1785–1793. You can view the statement at the website of the American College of Sports Medicine (ACSM): www.acsm.org/publications/pdf/FemaleAthlete.pdf.
2. Ibid., p. 1786.
3. Ibid.
4. William D. McArdle, Frank I. Katch, and Victor L. Katch. *Essentials of Exercise Physiology,* second edition (Philadelphia: Lippincott Williams & Wilkins, 2000), p. 77.
5. American College of Sports Medicine. *ACSM's Guidelines for Exercise Testing and Prescription,* sixth edition (Philadelphia: Lippincott Williams & Wilkins, 2000), p. 230.
6. Ibid., p. 253.
7. L. D. Zwiren. "Exercise Testing and Prescription Considerations Throughout Childhood." In American College of Sports Medicine. *ACSM's Resource Manual for Guidelines for Exercise Testing and Prescription,* fourth edition (Philadelphia: Lippincott Williams & Wilkins, 2001), table 60.1, p. 521.
8. American College of Sports Medicine. *ACSM's Guidelines for Exercise Testing and Prescription,* sixth edition (Philadelphia: Lippincott Williams & Wilkins, 2000), p. 225.
9. J. A. Buckwalter and N. E. Lane. "Athletics and Osteoarthritis." *Am J Sports Med* 25 (1997), pp. 873–881.
10. J. S. Skinner, "Chronic Fatigue Syndrome: Matching Exercise to Symptom Fluctuation." *The Physician and Sportsmedicine* 32 (2004), pp. 28–32.

Chapter 10: The Integrated Life

1. Eckhart Tolle. *The Power of Now: A Guide to Spiritual Enlightenment* (Novato, Calif: New World Library, 1999), p. 168.
2. Ibid., p. 98.
3. Wendy Palmer. *The Intuitive Body: Aikido as a Clairsentient Practice* (Berkeley, Calif: North Atlantic Books, 1995), p. 15.
4. Sharon Waxman. "From Imelda Marcos's Flats to the Golden Arches." *The New York Times* (January 24, 2004), p. A27. *People* magazine (February 9, 2004), p. 114.
5. Ibid.
6. R. Manning. "The Oil We Eat." *Harper's Magazine* (February 2004), pp. 37–45.
7. Jane E. Brody. "The Widening of America, or How Size 4 Became Size 0." *The New York Times* (January 20, 2004), p. D7.

8. David Hochman. "Food for Holiday Thought: Eat Less, Live to 140?" *The New York Times* (November 23, 2003), section 9, p. 1.

9. Peter Carey and Mark Emmons. "Focus Is on Firm That Aids Athletes." *San Jose Mercury News* (October 12, 2003), p. 1H.

10. T. L. Schwenk and C. D. Costley. "When Food Becomes a Drug: Nonanabolic Nutritional Supplement Use in Athletes." *Am J Sports Med* 30 (2002), pp. 907–916.

11. William D. McArdle, Frank I. Katch, and Victor L. Katch. *Essentials of Exercise Physiology,* second edition (Philadelphia: Lippincott Williams & Wilkins, 2000), p. 74.

12. Ibid., p. 56.

13. Charles Yesalis and Michael Bahrke. "Where There Is a Will to Gain an Edge, Athletes Find a Way." *The New York Times* (March 7, 2004), p. 9.

14. Kate Zernike. "Food Fight: Is Obesity the Responsibility of the Body Politic?" *The New York Times* (November 9, 2003), p. WK3.

About the Author

W. JACKSON DAVIS is professor of ecology and evolution at the University of California, Santa Cruz (UCSC), where he teaches exercise physiology. He is a certified health and fitness instructor of the American College of Sports Medicine and serves as strength and conditioning coach in the UCSC Athletic Department, where he trains athletes in IBC and prepares them for their individual sports. He has published more than 150 scientific papers, books, reviews, op-ed pieces, and articles. He received the Humboldt Award from Germany for outstanding original scientific research in the neurosciences.